MEDICAL PRACTICE CHANGE MANAGEMENT

Strategies and Techniques for the Changing Business of Healthcare

MEDICAL PRACTICE CHANGE MANAGEMENT

Strategies and Techniques for the Changing Business of Healthcare

PETER D. LUCASH

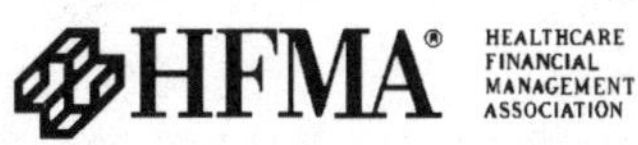

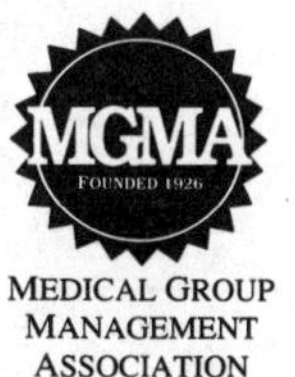

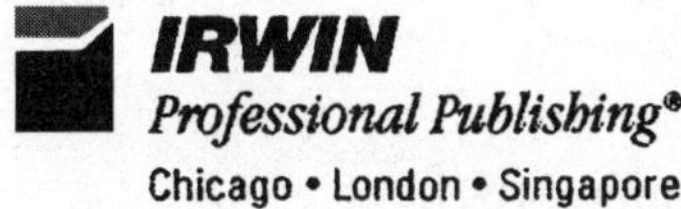

MEDICAL PRACTICE CHANGE MANAGMENT

Copyright © 1997 by Healthcare Financial Management Association. All rights reserved. Printed in the United States of America. Except as permitted under the United States Copyright Act of 1976, no part of this publication may be reproduced or distributed in any form or by any means, or stored in a data base or retrieval system, without the prior written permission of the publisher.

This publication is designed to provide accurate and authoritative information in regard to the subject matter covered. It is sold with the understanding that neither the author or the publisher is engaged in rendering legal, accounting, or other professional service. If legal advice or other expert assistance is required, the services of a competent professional person should be sought.

From a Declaration of Principles jointly adopted by a Committee of the American Bar Association and a Committee of Publishers.

2 3 4 5 6 7 8 9 0 DOC DOC 9 0 9 8 7

ISBN 0–7863–0998–9

Library of Congress Cataloging-in-Publication Data

Lucash, Peter D.
Medical practice change management: strategies and techniques for the changing business of healthcare / Peter D. Lucash.
p. cm.
Includes index.
ISBN 0–7863–0998–9
1. Medicine—Practice—United States. 2. Managed care plans (Medical care)—United States. I. Title.
R728.L826 1997
362.1'068—dc21 96–45342
http: / / www.mhcollege.com

Dedication

For Deborah,
my wife of nine years, my best friend for ten.
Truly the love of my life, the person I turn to
for advice, for support, and to listen.
Believe me when I tell you,
none of this would be possible without her.

ACKNOWLEDGMENTS

I'm sure that book editors are never amazed at the naiveté of authors. I've written a lot of things in my life—but a book is truly a whole new undertaking and puts a whole new meaning into the word "writer." Just as I gained a profound respect for teachers after the first time I taught a course, the time invested in writing this book gave me a profound sense of respect for those who undertake to write, edit, and publish books. This has been an adventure.

The trail to this writing is convoluted and is in many ways the result of many of the coincidences, chance encounters, timing, divine intervention, and kismet that make our lives what they are. Like many of my healthcare colleagues, my career has been somewhat nomadic, moving from place to place in response to the changing winds of the marketplace. Settled in comfortably at Montefiore Hospital in Pittsburgh, my family was dealt a blow when the hospital was sold one Saturday morning in October 1989. By March, the entire management team, including myself, was gone. Seeing that the opportunities in healthcare were changing, I eventually landed as the administrator of a specialty physician group in the Hudson Valley of New York State. In 1994, we left the northeast for Charleston, SC, where I renewed Lucash & Company.

An ad in *Modern Healthcare* led me to Jerry Kaye, the founder of Business Network. Jerry had the faith in me and supported me as I learned how to present a seminar. I am grateful for his support, faith and guidance, and the opportunity he gave me. I've been traveling with Business Network for two years now and am indebted to the many great people who schedule us, book our flights, ship our books, and generally try to keep us safe and comfortable while on the road. Mary Rose McKee, Sheila Higney, Jeannie Miller, Aimee Sanders, and Dee Pankow among others are in the current cast of characters who staff Business Network since becoming part of Irwin. The hundreds who have been to my seminars have sharpened my knowledge, challenged me, offered information, and, in some cases, offered solid advice. I have enjoyed and appreciated them all.

Kris Rynne, the editor at Irwin Professional Publishing who supported the idea for this book, and has become a friend over the time it has taken to write it. Kris has a talent for the right words and good advice, and generally makes the task of writing less daunting. She is a *great* editor. Of course, there is "Jimmy the Squirrel" who "encouraged" me.

My professional life and skills have been shaped by a number of key people who I've had the pleasure to work with and for over the years: Bernie Fuss, my mentor at Brookdale Hospital Medical Center in Brooklyn, NY: Keith Kinnally at HANYS, and at Montefiore, Irv Goldberg, Kip Goldberg, and Bill Youngblood; and in New York, Kathy Bozony and Beth Texter. Through all this, there are several people who have been my colleagues and friends and have made healthcare fun: Alan Green, Chuck Kaufman, Dan Berger, and Bob Tell, to name a few. My interest in healthcare grew from several places including: my Uncle, Dr. Herman Denber, who always told me I should write a book, and the men and women of the Spring Hill Community Ambulance Corps in Spring Valley, NY (all volunteers) with whom I spent six years and answered over 300 emergency calls.

In Charleston, I have been fortunate to work with Dr. Len Heere. I hope that I have served him well in some of his endeavors. In Charleston, a number of people have been very supportive, among these: Michael Abidor, then executive director of the Charleston Jewish Federation; the people of Synagogue Emanu-el; Lawrence Laddaga, an attorney who is currently present-elect of the South Carolina chapter of the HFMA; Kit Rogers of the Small Business Resource Center; and Kathleen Cartland of the Chamber of Commerce. At the College of Charleston, Dean Howard Rudd has been a friend and supporter, and the Associates of the Center for Entrepreneurship have been a source of professional friendship and learning, including Charles Cathcart, Richard Von Werssowetz, Bob Nagy, and Dave Drescher. A special thanks to Entrepreneur-in-Residence Stanley Foster Reed (coincidentally, also an Irwin author of *The Art of M&A*), who introduced me to the good people at the College and has been a supporter and friend.

For Jo Dee Massena—"Heads, Carolina." For the people at the USAir Club; for Starbuck's Coffee; "All Things Considered" the WSCI and WEZL radio stations; and Dilbert. Also, thanks to

Andrew and Elka Bernstein; Andrew threatened to stop talking to me until I finished the book. For beaches and waterfront around Charleston.

For my parents, who have always been there for me; my brother, Ricki; my in-laws, Dan and Adrienne Goldstein; my Aunt Sylvia and my late Uncle Lou, who've been with me and now my family since the beginning; my dear late grandmother, Bessie Goldenberg.

And especially for my children, Ellie and Aaron, who make me laugh, understand my absence, and talk with me when I'm away, and who are full of fun and play and questions—they are the joy of life.

As part of the alliance between HFMA and MGMA, these two Associations have collaborated in the review of this text. Both organizations recognize that change is the way of life of healthcare. The author for this book reflects on the changes taking place in medical practice management, which is an integral part of today's healthcare delivery system. In keeping with each Board's commitment to diversification, we are proud of this collaboration on this book and hope you enjoy reading it.

Richard L. Clarke, FHFMA
President and CEO
HFMA

Thomas L. Adams, CAE
Executive Vice President/CEO
MGMA

CONTENTS

Introduction

It's the end of the world as we know it.

R.E.M.

I recently met a surgeon, in practice for 34 years, who told me that he had just decided to retire. Actually, he decided to quit. He made this decision during a phone call with a utilization review nurse from an insurance company. My friend's patient had a mole that was suspected to be a basal cell carcinoma. He wanted to remove the mole and then send it for a biopsy—all in one procedure. The nurse was arguing that my friend should do a biopsy, wait for the lab results to come back, and then, at a second visit, remove the mole if necessary. He finally told her, "I don't care whether you pay for this or not. I'm doing one procedure on this patient, and then I'm quitting!"

This book is about revolutionary change—a complete rendering asunder of how healthcare services are organized, financed, and delivered. It is a story of an industry that is at once local and national. An industry that is at once coalescing and diverging, cooperating and fighting. There are no rules. There are attitudes, ways to think, and ways to look at things. In the end, it comes down to being very prepared and always ready to move, dodge, duck, hit the floor, dust yourself off, and start moving again.

This change is a revolution in the shift in power—a shift from the physician to the payer. The payers have now inserted themselves between the physician's stethoscope and the patient's skin, observing, approving of, and disapproving of the actions and decisions of the physicians. Payers have taken the position that they are responsible for providing for quality healthcare services for their customers, who they now call "members."

> What's that popping sound? It's a paradigm shifting.
>
> *Dilbert*

This book is written to help you manage your organization through the turmoil, to separate out fact from fiction, reality from paranoid delusions, assertive management from withdrawal and defeat. In my travels around this country, speaking to physicians, practice managers, dentists, podiatrists, physical therapists, and other "providers," I have found that people are hungry for information and help in running their practices. I also have found that people are angry, frustrated, defeated, outraged, and burning out. They often feel as though they are a high wire act in a dark tent, trying to maintain balance and move forward, all without any light and without a safety net underneath. I once commented to a chief executive officer (CEO) I worked for that I felt like I was walking through a minefield—one false step and KABOOM!!

As fast as the power shifts, it shifts again. What is the role of a physician? We venerate and long for the days of the family doctor who made house calls and treated the whole family—the "Dr. Welby" model. From there we have moved to a "specialist model," where specialists are the focus of care. I've even seen communities where the primary care physicians don't bother to have hospital admitting privileges. As this is written, we are moving through a stage where managed care plans are driving care, by intervening in treatment decisions, directing drugs to be used, time in a hospital, and the number and kind of referrals for specialty care. Even as we are moving through that stage, we are moving into a stage where control is shifting back to the providers. Large employers and employer groups are bypassing the managed care plans, contracting directly with providers, often through physician–hospital consortiums. These consortiums receive a pool of funds and in turn decide how to manage and divvy up the funds to pay for care. With the control of funds in the hands of the providers, control of medical decisions—the spending of the monies—returns to the providers. With this control comes the responsibility for utilization management and quality of care, taking back the responsibilities that managed care plans have usurped.

This book is written to encourage physicians to keep fighting the good fight. It is written so that good, dedicated physicians don't throw in the towel out of their frustration of dealing with a world that is very different from the one that they entered when they began to practice. Over my 18 years in healthcare, I have never seen such a period of upheaval and turmoil—an upheaval that reaches past the organization and into the personal psyche of the people who care for patients every day. Ours are very noble professions. There is a very strong ethic of commitment to patients, a commitment that transcends position, status, and power. What is palpable today, however, is a sense of disorientation, of frustration, of defeat. Battered by an increasing barrage of criticism from pundits, corporate chieftains, the media, insurance companies, and some for-profit chains, providers are being told that they are the "bad guys"—greedy, self-centered, often inept, and aloof.

> Only the paranoid survive.
>
> *Andy Grove, CEO, Intel Corp.*

An apt observation. It is a very different world out there. My uncle, a retired physician, tells the parable: "If the federal government had its way, you would get a shot when you were born. You would be perfectly healthy until age 65, and then you would drop dead."

Patients are dealing with new forms of health insurance that they don't fully understand—not that they understand the traditional indemnity plans either. The penalties for this lack of understanding can be severe. There is a great deal of information and misinformation, if not disinformation, leading to feelings of confusion and frustration that often are vented on the physicians and their staffs, who have their own set of problems.

Ours is a nation that has grown a health insurance system that is tied to employment. In the traditional world of indemnity healthcare insurance, the employer would select a health insurance plan for its employees and pay all or most of the premiums, which were deductible to the employer. Armed with their healthcare insurance cards (jokingly referred to as "health Mastercards") employees could then go out and choose any provider from anywhere in the country, and the health plan would pay the provider or reimburse the employee based upon the provisions of the benefit package the employer had purchased.

That has all changed. The cost of healthcare has captured the attention of politicians, corporate chieftains, chief financial officers, Wall Street investors, and the average citizen. Pick up a newspaper or magazine, and there is likely to be an article about the cost of healthcare. In his first book, "Iacocca," former Chrysler Corporation chairman Lee Iacocca noted that he spent more per car on employee healthcare insurance than he spent on steel. A powerful image. (Of course, that begs the question whether it's a comment on the quality of Chrysler products!) In 1995, AT&T spent $1 billion—20 percent of its profits—on healthcare coverage. In 1996, AT&T sent 100,000 managers and dependents into managed care plans. All through the 1980s and into the 1990s, healthcare spending has been rising at rates that are several times the increase in the consumer price index. By any measure, costs are a major burden. Change in healthcare is being driven by large corporations and modern management techniques. Modern management calls for moving away from an autocratic, dictatorial style—such as managed care organizations (MCOs) directing treatment—toward a model where organizations of providers band together, and the organization takes on the role of coach and cheerleader, pushing the physicians toward doing a better job, and demonstrating *how* they can do a better job. Different attitude—better outcome.

Healthcare is a very complex process. It is a process that must be simplified in order to be more efficient, more effective, and to demonstrate that we are accomplishing something. It is no longer acceptable for us to hide behind a mysterious world of linguistic shorthand, scientific terms, lab tests, and large technology-driven equipment. Employers, patients, and payers are demanding that the mystery be removed, that we be able to demonstrate that the money being spent accomplishes something. We often have wondered why treatment practices vary so much from community to community. We now are demanding that we search for the "best practices." Valid questions are being asked: Why does utilization vary so much across the country? Business is asking the hard questions: Why is the process so complicated? Modern management has learned that the more complex the process, the more prone it is to error.

So we look for ways to measure outcomes and quality of care, ways to say who is doing a good job and who is not doing so good a job. Some measures are rudimentary, such as patient satisfaction. Others are crude: mortality rates, adverse events, utilization rates. For the first time, physicians are gaining access to data and information that compare their practices and outcomes to the practices and outcomes of other physicians. By doing so, physicians can look at what they do individually and move towards the "best" methods. The utilization management of today remains an authoritarian, disciplinarian model, one where the decisions appear to be arbitrary and without regard to the needs of the individual patients. As physicians band together with hospitals into large groups responsible for the total care of the patients, including spending the insurance premiums, these groups can become the "coach" devising and sharing information as to the "best practices" and pushing physicians to innovate and develop the better ways to treat patients as effectively and as efficiently as possible. It is no longer simply a question of the lowest cost; we now demand evidence that what we do produces a result that we want.

There is, I believe, a resurgence of respect for physicians. The demand is for "less art, more science." As professionals, physicians' loyalties lie with their profession and their patients. Medicine is founded on a culture that is egalitarian in nature. It is a culture that honors collaboration and the sharing of advances, discoveries, and breakthroughs. Keeping pace with advances is difficult—there has been an explosion in the volume of data and information, as well as the sources of these advances. Because of the increasing complexity of clinical and business practices, physicians and other providers are banding together into larger organizations that make it possible to bring the "best practices" to the practice level. Solo and small groups have difficulty innovating and adapting the best practices; we need the depth of the larger organization in order to accomplish this.

The premise in writing this book is that the changes in healthcare impact all facets of the industry down to how paper is handled in the office. Physicians are facing a blizzard of market forces, conflicting prognostications and advice, and enormous uncertainty as to what their options are and what they should do. Many react blindly while others are paralyzed by inaction. In this book, I focus on the forces at play, the players involved (how they are motivated, how they think), and how physicians can position themselves to build the future for their practices and their personal goals.

Many a tree has been felled in the cloud of information and misinformation about managed care and managing under managed care (or, may I suggest, managing *with* managed care). Let me let you in on a little secret—managed care is really pretty simple. There are some fundamentals. *Managed care is all in the fundamentals—and it's all fundamental!* Focus on the fundamentals, and you'll be fine.

In writing this book, the approach that I've taken is a comprehensive, practical approach to developing and implementing strategies and techniques for medical practices to manage in the "new healthcare" arena. The chapters, you will note, mostly take a micro approach, focusing on techniques to be used on a daily basis. Chapter 8 on strategy and, to some extent, Chapter 9 on marketing take a macro viewpoint, offering the strategic options for practices. In the appendixes, I have included a variety of references and resources for your use, including a medical practice business plan workbook, a glossary, a list of useful web sites on the Internet, and management resources.

Healthcare is different from any other business—it needs a soul. This book is written to help you run well and keep your soul. Keep up the good fight!

1

CHAPTER

The New Players

We are undergoing the greatest upheaval in the organization, financing, and delivery of healthcare that we have ever experienced. Roles and responsibilities are changing and being shifted around. There are a host of new players in the healthcare arena, splitting off parts of patients' bodies and parts of their care. The management of the premium dollar is shifting from the health plans to the large provider groups, which are in turn acting as insurance companies—and taking out the requisite state insurance company licenses. Healthcare has moved to center stage in the political arena and has influenced the outcome of national elections. Healthcare spending in 1994 grew to $949.4 billion, or 13.7 of the gross national product (GNP), and has the attention of the top management of large corporations. Wall Street sees healthcare as a major expense for corporations, as well as a major source of opportunity to exploit economies of scale, integration, and management synergies.

What has changed more than anything is the orientation of power. Physicians were traditionally the "captain" of the healthcare team. They were the only ones with the power to prescribe treatments, many of which were carried out by nurses, pharmacists, physical therapists, or others. Since World War II, indemnity health insurance plans have increasingly paid part of the fees for physician services, often close to the full fee that was charged. Medicare and Medicaid removed or lowered financial barriers to accessing medical care for millions of people.

Managed care plans changed this dynamic. With traditional indemnity plans, employees can go to any provider, any time, anywhere. In choosing a provider, people will look to neighbors, friends, and fellow employees. Perhaps they have seen an ad or know of someone who has used a particular physician. Or, they simply follow the directive of a physician telling them "We'll make an appointment with Dr. X." Under managed care plans, however, the plan defines the universe of choices. All services must be authorized and approved by the patient's primary care physician (PCP); this person guards and controls the gate to all other services and hence has been given the title of "gatekeeper." Many plans also require that some or all services be approved by the plan's utilization management reviewer. In either event, the goal is to control access, limit the universe of choices, and limit utilization of all services except primary medical care. By doing so, managed care plans can reduce utilization, thereby reducing costs, and thereby reducing the premiums charged to employers.

While indemnity plans had a contractual relationship only with the employer, managed care plans take a broader view. In return for lower premiums, the plans will define the universe of providers from which patients can select. To do that, the plans must provide for the network of providers, and to do so, they must contract with the providers necessary to cover the scope of services called for in the contract. For physicians and other providers, the fundamental difference is that there is now a contractual relationship between the plan and the provider. No contract, no service.

In Figure 1-1, the "new relationships" among the covered lives, buyers (usually employers), payers, and providers is presented. "Covered lives" is an insurance term referring to the beneficiaries of an insurance policy, in this case, the employees or retirees and their respective dependents. As discussed above, the health plan now has contractual relationships with all of the providers who will be providing services for the plan members.

FIGURE 1–1

The New Relationships

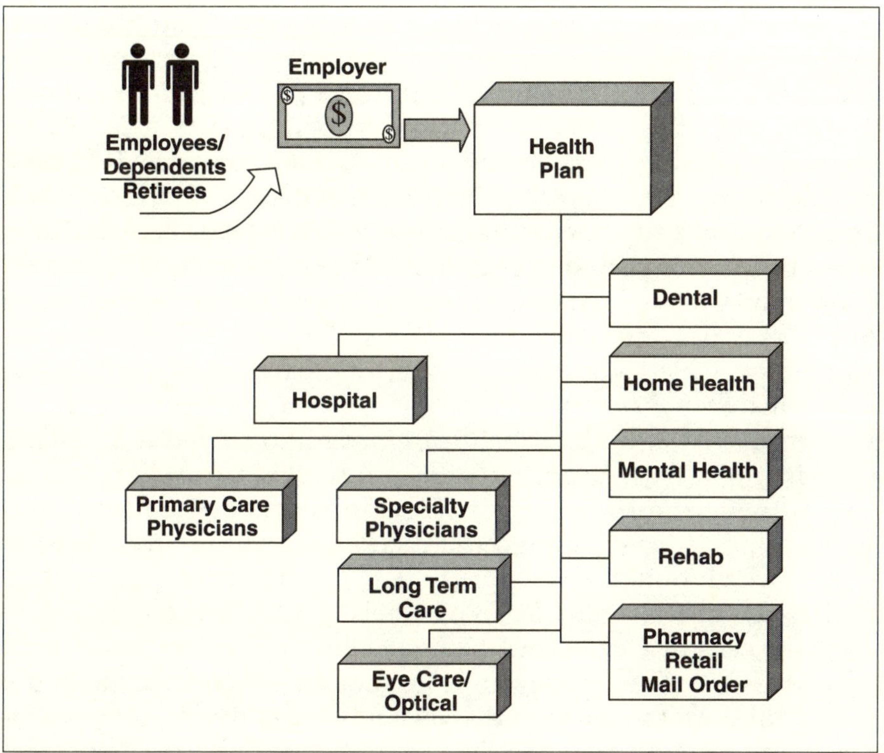

Many Blue Cross plans have had contracts with hospitals for many years. These contracts typically were somewhat limited in scope, addressing the computation of rates and the filing and auditing of cost reports. Provider contracts with managed care plans, however, are much more comprehensive in scope in defining the business relationship between the payer and the providers.

The story is told of a group of physicians on a bus tour. Midway through the trip, one of the passengers stands up, grabs his chest, and falls to the floor. One of the physicians stands up and announces, "I'm an internist, and I think he has indigestion. I'll take care of him!" A cardiologist stands up and announces, "No, it's a heart problem. I'll take care of him!" The bus driver then stops the bus, turns off the engine, turns to the passengers and calmly says, "My bus, my patient."

In the face of the rising dominance of payers and the financing of health care services, there is a shake out underway among the payers. In 1994, Travelers and Metropolitan Life Insurance merged their group health insurance operations to form a new company named MetraHealth. Less than a year later, however, MetraHealth was taken over by United Healthcare. United Healthcare, already one of the largest managed care companies in the country, was poised to leap to number one by winning a hotly contested battle to buy Wellpoint, the managed care subsidiary of Blue Cross of California. It was not to happen, however, as the merger unraveled a few months later in the face of two chief executive officers who couldn't complete the agreement. As this is written, Aetna and U.S. Healthcare have announced a merger, a combination that will create the largest health insurer in the country. Anthem, the Blue Cross licensee in Indiana, Kentucky, and part of Illinois, has announced a merger with Blue Cross of New Jersey, which only a week earlier had announced a merger with Blue Cross of Delaware. Keeping track of all this is like trying to track the card in a three-card Monte game.

The rise of the payers has generated a new corollary: the merger of the financing and delivery functions. By and large, managed care organizations (MCO) do not deliver care—they must contract with physicians, hospitals, and other providers to provide the services that the payers have contracted to pay for with the employers and employees. Unlike traditional indemnity plans, the health plan product is not only the scope of services covered, but the network of providers who actually provide the service. In some markets, MCOs have set up "captive" physician groups. These groups contract with a plan to provide services, typically primary care services, for plan members exclusively. Health plans often are barred from employing physicians directly under state corporate practice of medicine laws—laws that forbid nonphysicians or nonphysician corporations from owning part of a medical practice or employing physicians. By setting up a long term contractual arrangement, the benefits to the health plan of ownership and control can be garnered while still remaining at arm's length from the physicians. In some instances, the plan will provide management services for the groups as well, also under a contractual arrangement (see the discussion of management services organizations below).

Not only have today's health plans taken on the responsibility of providing for a provider network themselves, some employers are returning to the historic practice of some industries. In Pittsburgh, South Side Hospital is located across from the old Jones and Laughlin (J&L) Steel plant. In the olden days of the hospital, there was a "J&L" floor, staffed by J&L physicians, to care for the company's workers and dependents. In the same tradition, Kaiser Steel, Southern California Electric and Gas, and John Deere have established corporate health clinics. John Deere (makers of tractors, farm equipment, and other such goods) originally set up clinics to provide care for its employees in medically underserved, rural areas near their plants. Approached by other firms looking for medical services, Deere took them on. Deere eventually started John Deere Health Plan, marketing managed care and indemnity products throughout the Midwest.

We now are seeing a developing trend that further consolidates power, authority, and responsibility for healthcare services. The move in some markets, notably Southern California, is toward "global capitation." In a global capitation scheme, the premium dollars flow from the employer through a health plan to a "super" provider entity. This super provider entity, which could be a large physician group, a physician–hospital organization (PHO), a hospital, or whatever, is then responsible for managing the finances and, most importantly, paying all other providers down the food chain: hospitals, all physicians, rehab services, mental health, and so on. In some instances, employers are contracting directly with these super provider entities. As will be discussed in Chapter 4, "Capitation," when a super provider entity takes on a risk contract directly with an employer, the provider entity is then acting as an insurance company and must be licensed by the state. The net result is that there are now providers becoming insurance companies, so that there are insurance companies providing direct care again, which is contrary to the pattern of contracted networks that has driven the growth of managed care in the past 10 years. Yes, in health care, it takes a scorecard.

Part of the healthcare revolution involves the way in which the industry has organized itself. In response to changing needs and opportunities, new kinds of organizations are being created. In the next few pages, we will discuss some of the more important ones.

MANAGED CARE ORGANIZATIONS (MCO)

Managed care organization (MCO) is the generic term for any kind of organization that provides health insurance coverage to a population and, further, imposes requirements for utilization management to control the quality of certain, defined services. There are a myriad of varieties of MCOs, from the traditional health maintenance organization (HMO), to the preferred provider organization (PPO), to direct contracting networks, and so on. The variations on managed care are limited only by the limitations of the human imagination.

HEALTH MAINTENANCE ORGANIZATIONS (HMO)

Health maintenance organizations, known as HMOs, are the granddaddy of all managed care. The original HMOs were known as "prepaid health plans." HMOs such as the Kaiser Health Plan, the Health Insurance Plan of Greater New York (the HIP Plan), and Group Health of Puget Sound took on the responsibility for the delivery of all the services that a patient required. In return for the insurance premium (the "prepaid"), these plans also would provide the care. Unlike most health insurance plans, there also were low or no copayments and deductibles. A further major difference was that the plans employed their own physicians either directly or through an exclusive contract. This is what is known as a "staff model" HMO. (In a number of states, certain entities, such as hospitals and HMOs *can* employ physicians.) Finally, these plans were organized as not-for-profit organizations.

What makes HMOs different from other forms of managed care is that they share a portion of the underwriting risk of financing healthcare services with some of the providers who provide the care. The sharing of risk is what makes HMOs different from other types of MCOs. It is this sharing of risk that defines HMOs as carrying on an insurance function—in fact, they are insurance companies. As a result, HMOs are licensed by the state insurance department and, in some states, they also may be required to be licensed or otherwise registered with the state health department.

In addition to the assumption of risk, the key element of an HMO is ongoing preventative care to prevent serious illnesses and, therefore, expenses. The old line HMOs, such as the Kaiser Plan, were founded on the theory of prepaid care with a focus on preventative care. The underlying theory is this:

1. Every patient has a "family physician," in the traditional model, who is responsible for all health care. This physician is expected to know the patient, coordinate all of the patient's care, and help the patient to remain healthy.
2. The HMO will encourage patients to seek advice and treatment from their family physicians by paying for all services, including those which indemnity plans do not pay for, such as routine checkups, screening exams (such as mammograms and pap smears), and immunizations.
3. The combination of one family physician and preventative care will lead to fewer illnesses and the need for fewer expensive services, particularly hospitalization.

To support this, there is a sharing of financial risk between the insurer (HMO) and the providers. This sharing of risk occurs either through a capitation payment mechanism or a "risk withhold" mechanism (see Chapter 3, "Changes in Reimbursement," for a discussion of all this). In order to enforce the utilization controls, HMOs utilize the primary care physicians as "gatekeepers." The role of the gatekeeper is exactly as the name implies, much like the green man at the doors leading to the Emerald City. Gatekeepers are the primary care physicians, which include internists, family practice physicians, pediatricians, and gynecologists (sometimes). HMO members can always go to their primary care physician (PCP), but the PCP must approve all other services by making a referral. (More on this later.)

The first true HMO was the Kaiser Health Plan. Originally founded by Kaiser Steel to care for shipyard workers building Liberty Ships during World War II, it evolved into one of the largest such organizations in the world. Kaiser is actually three organizations: Kaiser Health Plan, Kaiser Hospitals, and the Permanente Medical Group. Kaiser was the first of the "closed panel" HMOs, which employ their own physicians. In its historic California market, care for Kaiser members was provided by Permanente Medical Group employee physicians, who virtually served only served Kaiser members. Patients needing admission to a hospital were admitted to a Kaiser hospital, got their prescriptions at Kaiser pharmacies, and so on. Kaiser served its members within its own world—it was the first integrated network.

As Kaiser expanded its geographic reach, opening up in New York, Washington, D.C., North Carolina, Cleveland, and other cities and states, Kaiser moved away from the closed panel to the "open panel." Open panel HMOs use networks of physicians in the community who serve HMO and non-HMO patients alike. The advantage of the open panel is that the HMO organization does not have to build all of the infrastructure necessary to provide the scope of benefit services.

Building an infrastructure is a "build," "buy," or "lease" decision. To "build" means to develop the resources internally by hiring staff, buying equipment, building buildings, and such. To "buy" means to acquire the necessary resources through a purchase of an existing organization or pieces of one or more organizations. In a "lease" decision, a company uses and pays for only those resources it needs from a supplier. In the "open staff" model, HMOs "lease" the services of the providers, paying for that portion of the supplier's (provider's) capacity and infrastructure that it needs. The supplier bears the risk and responsibility for building sufficient resources to meet the needs of the HMO. Capital invested in the HMO can be directed toward marketing and supporting other cash flow requirements as the plan is built.

As more HMOs were created, spurred by the federal HMO act of 1973, the newer HMOs evolved away from the staff model. Instead, the newer HMOs chose the faster growth strategy of leasing the providers they needed. Since the newer HMOs did not have to build all of the infrastructure, the newer HMOs needed less capital to enter the business and could grow faster; if they needed more capacity to deliver services, they would contract with more local providers. Combining this evolution with the federal law that mandated that employers with 25 or more employees offer an HMO health insurance option if an HMO was available in a market began to generate the rapid growth of HMOs and managed care in the United States.

PREFERRED PROVIDER ORGANIZATIONS (PPO)

Preferred provider organizations (PPOs) were the first competitors of HMOs. PPOs work differently than HMOs: the focus of a PPO is the delivery of pure economic incentives to its members through discounted pricing, with no sharing of risk. PPO organizations develop a network of providers in a market area who agree to a lower fee schedule in return for access to the patient roster. The PPO plan offers its full benefits to members who utilize the network—the "preferred providers." However, if members choose to go out of the network and use a "nonpreferred" provider, they will not receive the full value of their benefits. The plan may pay up to what it pays a network provider, or even reduce that amount in reimbursement to the member. In essence, the PPO is a giant discounted fee network.

A new twist on PPOs is an unfortunate one—one dubbed "silent PPOs." Silent PPOs are companies that build the provider network, but rather than contracting with employers, they simply assign, or lease, the provider agreement to an indemnity carrier that may currently be paying providers full or near full fee. Providers have signed a contract expecting to get a new source of patients, when in fact there was never any intent of that happening. In many contracts, there is a provision known as an "assignment" clause. This clause allows the PPO to assign the contract and its provisions to another party. A reasonable basis for this provision is in the event that the PPO or HMO is sold to another payer organization, or a provider sells or merges with another organization. All existing provider contracts could be transferred over to the new organization without the need to sign hundreds of new contracts. The silent PPO abuses this, however. The rate the provider has agreed to is transferred to a payer for whom the provider may already have a contract, or to one with which the provider would not agree to the same terms or conditions.

POINT OF SERVICE PLANS

One of the major marketing problems facing an HMO is the restriction of choice of providers. PPOs offer an advantage to members in that they can self-refer out of the network, albeit with a financial penalty. An HMO usually will not pay for out-of-plan care absent a true life-threatening emergency. In response to this competition, the point of service, or POS, plans were created. POS plans combine the best features of an HMO, risk contracting and the primary care physician as gatekeeper, with the ability of the member to self-refer out of the network with the financial penalty. Since utilization is not completely under the control of the HMO, the premiums for these plans are higher than those for a standard HMO.

PHYSICIAN–HOSPITAL ORGANIZATIONS (PHO)

Physician–hospital organizations (PHOs) are the latest fad in the everlasting effort of hospitals to align their interests with those of their physicians. You may remember the 1980s, when *the* hot topic for hospitals was "physician bonding." Recognizing that only physicians can admit patients, hospitals literally tripped over themselves in vain, and usually futile, attempts to influence the referral decisions being made in the physician's office. Hospitals did everything from offering free and close-in parking and free practice management consulting to forming joint ventures, inviting physicians to invest in high technology equipment, such as CT scanners and MRIs, as well as in medical office buildings located next to the hospital. Driven by the desire for economic gain by all parties concerned, hospitals plunged into all sorts of "diversification" activities. Some built medical office buildings. Some bought office buildings. Some opened restaurants, others, health clubs, and one I know had the Pepsi vending machine franchise, installed private phone systems, managed the local country club, and maintained the local race track. Most of the ventures failed miserably.

Since their introduction, PHOs have evolved in a very different direction. Unlike their medical staff hospital (MeSH) ancestors, PHOs are sticking to the health field. In most cases, the principal reason for organizing a PHO has been to align the interests of the hospital, primary care physicians, and specialty physicians in order to solicit managed care contracts. The rationale is that in order to truly lower hospital utilization, it is necessary for the medical staff to be committed to this pattern of practice. The PHO organization enables the three parties—hospitals, primary care physicians, and specialty physicians—to coordinate and jointly plan their efforts and share in the financial rewards by reducing utilization.

The typical structure of a PHO is an equally shared ownership between the hospital and the participating members of the medical staff. The board of directors is typically also equally shared. In order to be a member of the PHO, the physicians must invest hard cash into the PHO corporation. To avoid antitrust and fraud and abuse issues, the money that is invested must truly be "at risk" of being lost if the investment is not successful. The returns on the investment (ROI) also must be tied to financial performance and not to the number and/or quality of referrals made into the PHO. Payments to the provider investors that are related to the quality or quantity of referrals would be deemed a "kickback," which could be a felony.

As with any managed care plan, *the* critical component is the ability to control utilization. If you can't control utilization, you can't control cost. And if you can't control cost, you can't crank down the premiums and you can't compete in the market. Remember: MCOs, as with all insurance plans, exist in a competitive marketplace trying to sell a product—health insurance coverage—to employers. To be successful, the MCO must offer a plan that is comprehensive in scope and one that buyers (employers) will perceive as providing value for their premium dollar. Note that I say "value" as opposed to "lowest cost." If the competition down the street charges $50 less for each "thing" that he does, but he does three times as many things as you do, the MCO is not getting any benefit—it makes more sense to get better value by contracting with you than with the competitor who appears to be cheaper.

PHOs are beginning to further evolve, taking on additional and related functions. In particular, they are beginning to provide management services such as billing, financial management, and the like. What is very interesting to observe is that physicians are trusting hospitals to manage sensitive functions which they previously kept very private. The PHO organizations are founded on the premise of a joint venture between the hospital and its medical staff, a joint venture based upon financial needs and mutual strategic goals. In that sense, PHOs offer a sound business opportunity for all parties.

The jury is still out on PHOs. In theory, they make sense, as there is an alliance between the hospitals and the physicians in seeking out managed care contracts. In the "good old days," hospitals and physicians were often at odds. In the managed care world, it is in the mutual interests of hospitals and physicians to band together to seek MCO contracts, since each needs the other. Physicians can only admit to hospitals that also participate in a plan, and hospitals need their physicians to participate in order to admit patients.

INTEGRATED DELIVERY SYSTEMS (IDS)

Integrated delivery systems (IDS) are one of the many hot buzzwords floating through healthcare today—the "holy grail" of health care organization. The underlying concept of an IDS organization is to bring together all the provider types—hospitals, physicians, outpatient care, nursing homes, and such—into one organization. IDS organizations can manage full risk capitation contracts, and we are now seeing IDS organizations taking on the payer function as well. This is "one stop shopping" at its best. Employers need only go to one organization, and all their needs will be taken care of. In an increasing number of markets, we are seeing exactly that evolution; employers are bypassing the health plans and contracting with the providers. Through IDS and IDS-like organizations, this becomes very feasible.

The theory argues that there is a "mature" IDS, one that includes all of the ancillary services, post-acute and sub-acute care, and, most importantly, the insurance function as part of this creature. These self-contained universes, which can offer an employer/insurance buyer not only the insurance but all of the providers a patient could need, theoretically, through the integration vertically and horizontally of all aspects of production, can achieve the lowest cost. This notion, however, runs counter to the experience of the rest of the business, which has found that being all things to all people doesn't work too well. This is an age where companies are outsourcing various core functions. For example, airlines are outsourcing baggage handling and others are outsourcing their information systems or their mail and copying rooms. In such an age, one wonders if consolidating all these functions makes the best sense.

IDS organization theory argues that the pieces need to be related somehow. Some would argue that an IDS needs to be in one corporate structure, that is, that a holding company needs to own all of the pieces. Some of these arrangements may be through joint ventures with another organization. IDS organizations also can be "virtual" organizations, that is, they are tied together through contractual or other working agreements, but may lack common ownership.

What is critical to successful IDS organizations is the ability to move patient information. In an ideal world, a patient will be moved to the exactly appropriate level of care the instant his condition dictates. Since the IDS organization controls all of the parts, each part is always ready to provide the services that are needed. To accomplish this, the various component providers must be able to access up-to-date medical records instantly.

Information systems integration—the ability to move information among several organizations—has historically been hampered by incompatible computer systems that cannot share information. There are technical solutions, often expensive ones, that can overcome the incompatibility. A new force, however, is emerging as a solution: the Internet. A federally sponsored demonstration project in West Virginia is placing medical records on the Internet, enabling remote providers to access the record as needed.

One wonders whether there will ever be, or why there should be, true integrated delivery systems. If faced with a decision whether to become part of an IDS, evaluate carefully the goals of the organization, the governance structure, financial and information systems capacity, and the management team: in short, the fundamental elements of any successful business.

MANAGEMENT SERVICES ORGANIZATIONS (MSO) AND PHYSICIAN PRACTICE MANAGEMENT COMPANIES (PPMC)

Providing management services to medical practices is not a new concept. We are used to local bookkeeping services, payroll services, and billing services providing specialized functions. The expanded definition of management services organizations (MSOs) arose as investors saw medical practices as a business sector that could benefit from consolidation and economies of scale. This is a fast growing business sector, and several companies are publicly traded on the stock markets, such as MedPartners, InPhyMed, Phycor, and Caremark (which has been taken over by MedPartners). These companies are also being called physician practice management companies, or PPMC.

MSOs come in many sizes and shapes. They exist because nonphysicians generally cannot employ physicians, nor can nonphysicians invest in a physician practice. The physician (or "professional") corporation (P.C.) will sell to an MSO the hard assets of a practice. The P.C., then, remains as a shell, with no assets. The physicians remain as partners and/or employees. The P.C. then contracts with the MSO to provide all of the resources needed to run a practice other than the physicians themselves, including: facilities, equipment, staff, financial, billing and marketing services, and contracting with health plans. In some instances, the health plans contract with the MSO which in turn provides for the physician network through the practices managed by the MSO. These contracts are typically very long term, as much as 30 to 40 years in length. Since MSOs are not medical practices, the MSO can sell equity interests in the company to outside, nonphysician investors. Further, since many practices are being grouped together and managed as one central organization, there is a larger asset and financial base upon which to base leases, loans, purchasing power, and even contracts with managed care organizations.

One of the selling points of MSOs is contract negotiation and network development. MSOs can bring in professional staff to solicit and negotiate contracts with other MSOs. Hospital-based MSOs can develop their own networks, which, when combined with the hospital's independent medical staff, can either create an independent practice association (IPA) or a PHO, which can be a vehicle for MSO contracting.

Again, remember that medical practices must be bound together into some sort of corporate entity with other physicians in order for group contracting to work. The physicians must invest capital that is at risk in order for the practices to negotiate as a group with managed care plans. Otherwise, it is a conspiracy to fix prices, which is illegal.

Managing physicians' practices is one of the hot growth niche businesses in healthcare, and it has attracted Wall Street and venture capital monies. Physicians' practices are still dominated by small, or relatively small, independent organizations that can benefit from the economies of scale of larger organizations. Caremark, the troubled company convicted of paying kickbacks and assorted other violations of fraud and abuse statutes, has been transformed into an MSO, and then taken over by MedPartners. Phycor and MedPartners are just two startups that have been chasing the physician practice market.

> Managing physicians is like trying to herd cats!
>
> *Wall Street Analyst*

HOSPITALS

Fear not! There still will be hospitals. Pundits who claim that hospitals will disappear, become giant intensive care units, and so on, are far off the mark. First of all, the alternatives to hospitals are not well developed and suffer from intractable management problems, particularly in finding and, most especially, keeping qualified, honest staff. In smaller and rural areas, hospitals are the true linchpin of the healthcare services for a community, without which there isn't sufficient demand to support diagnostic services and professional staffs. Stand-alone emergency rooms are also of limited usefulness and are highly insufficient unless they can find other missions. Yes, average length of stay has dropped dramatically, leaving wings full of closed rooms, lacking any patients. In larger, over-bedded markets, hospitals will continue to close or merge with stronger institutions, closing beds and consolidating services. At the same time, advances in technology and treatment modalities enable physicians to treat more patients and to treat patients who once could not have withstood the rigors of the treatment of choice. At this writing, "window" heart surgery is being tried, where, rather than sawing through the sternum and opening the full chest to perform coronary bypass surgery, a small window is opened in the side of the patients' chest, and, working in a much smaller area than open chest surgery, the bypass work is done, leaving the patient much less traumatized and able to go home and to recover faster. Gallstone surgery is the classic example of this, once requiring a two-week stay in the hospital. With the advent of laparoscopic cholecystectomy, surgery is now performed through four small incisions in the abdomen. Although operatory time is slightly longer, patients are being discharged in about five days, and they are able to go back to work or resume their routine shortly thereafter. Lower cost and lower length of stay equals reduced bed need. But with the trauma of the surgery dramatically reduced, there is an expanded cohort of patients who can be safely operated on, who could not have withstood the rigors of the traditional surgery.

I believe that the hospital of the future will be the linchpin of the healthcare system of the future, merging hospital services, outpatient services, nursing home care, home care, and physicians. The "trend du jour" that has spread rapidly and is growing is the acquisition of physician practices by hospitals. We are seeing this in large and small hospitals, in urban and rural settings. Physicians are heading for the exit, and hospitals are moving into the ownership vacuum in order to protect themselves, as well as to fulfill their commitment to their community. By and large, I am not so sure that hospitals will create their own managed care plans, but they will succeed by focusing on what they know how to do—organize and deliver patient care.

ALTERNATIVE SITE PROVIDERS

Healthcare is undergoing two divergent trends: one is consolidation and the other is fragmentation, as companies are being created to carve out smaller and more defined niches in the care continuum. Within these niches, there are the inevitable attempts to then consolidate in order to achieve the economies of scale which are incompatible with the small markets being carved out by these companies. Technological advances are making it possible for more and more services to be safely moved out of the hospital and into homes and a variety of noninstitutional settings. These advances include advances in pharmaceuticals as well as the "heavy" technology of CT, MRI, and PET scanners. Advances in psychopharmaceuticals—drugs for the treatment of mental illness—have had a dramatic impact, enabling tens of thousands of patients in giant state psychiatric hospitals (often nothing more than large wards that have advanced very little from the asylum days) to be safely discharged into community settings. Although many of the patients no longer need to be hospitalized, they do need continual support in the community, from medical care to social activities to help with daily living, and it took many years before many of these systems were in place, albeit not in all communities. The chronically mentally ill are not a privately insured market, however, so we have not seen any of the private, for-profit psychiatric care companies going after management contracts to build hospitals to attract these patients.

Other examples of alternative site providers include: birthing centers, staffed by midwives and sometimes even owned by hospitals; freestanding ambulatory surgery centers, which were knocked out by hospital-based centers and anti-kickback and fraud and abuse regulations; and home health care agencies, which are experiencing expansion of the scope of services and niche markets such as pediatrics, psychiatric, and infusion therapy (e.g., chemotherapy). Infusion therapy services have been scarred by the kickbacks paid by companies such as Caremark (formerly part of Baxter International) and T2 Medical, among others.

All these new players came about as healthcare develops and matures as an industry. The new providers, new services, consolidations, mergers, acquisitions—healthcare is looking more and more like the rest of the business world.

The modern history of commerce and business traces back to the Middle Ages. Until that time, people were mostly self sufficient, growing their own food and making their own clothes, tools, and other goods that they needed. As towns and villages evolved, trade grew, and commerce was dominated by small "cottage" industries. From there, western civilization evolved into large centralized businesses, manufacturing goods in mass quantities. The rise of the mass merchant, Sears, Roebuck being among the first, began an era dominated by large, centralized organizations that are national or worldwide in scope. And so is it with health care. We've moved to the town stage and are moving into the stage of large, centralized organizations that are national in scope. These organizations have access to capital for investment, and they have the staying power to wage a competitive fight to achieve market share and presence.

Faced with a rapidly evolving market, the challenge before medical practices is to find a niche position where they can meet the needs of a customer or customers. In this book, I will be building the pieces toward constructing an action plan and business plan for a practice. The starting point is to build a market profile—who's doing what for whom and where.

Appendix D is a workbook for developing a medical practice business plan—part of the plan is an assessment of the market. For our discussion here, I'll focus on a certain point. The first step in building your plan for change is to compile data:

1. Define your market area: identify where your patients live and work by zip code and by county. Compile demographic data by age and sex.
2. Compile a list of all HMOs and PPOs currently licensed to operated in your market area. Note the counties or other geographic areas in which each is able to operate.
3. Compile key data on each plan:
   a. Number of members—Break out by commercial, Medicare, Medicaid.
   b. Number of physicians—Primary care and specialty.
4. List competitor practices in your market area:
   a. List practices and physician names.
   b. List locations: note which physicians practice at each location.
   c. Note any special services by location.
   d. List hospital affiliations.
   e. List HMO/PPO affiliations.

FIGURE 1–2

Four Stages of Managed Care

Stage 1: Under 20% HMO Penetration	Stage 2: 20–40% HMO Penetration

◆ Demands for lower provider prices
◆ Insurers have low volume of enrollees
◆ Payer base is fragmented
◆ Fee for service dominates
	◆ Demands for lower (still) provider prices
	  ◆ Focus on inpatient costs
	  ◆ Capitation growing
	◆ Insurer enrollees increasing
	◆ Moderately fragmented payer base
	◆ Providers beginning to consolidate

Stage 3: 40–60% HMO Penetration	**Stage 4: 60%+ HMO Penetration**
◆ Large insurers begin to control market ◆ Physician income declines ◆ Aggressive utilization management and controls; reduces tests, procedures	◆ Insurers consolidate to few; concentrated payer base ◆ Capitated pricing of providers increases ◆ Price war among HMOs, providers

Source: H.M. Roussel, *Living with Managed Care: A View From the Front* (Englewood, CO: Medical Group Management Association, 1996), p. 15.

5. List major employers by plant / facility location:
   a. Number of employees: managerial and hourly.
   b. Health plan(s) used and where the purchasing decision is made (local, nationally, or union contract fund).

Your goal through the process is to create a portrait of your market. One task is to assess the level of managed care in your market. There are various schemes around, the most common I've seen is a four-stage rating system (Figure 1-2).

With the market portrait completed, you then move on to collecting the data to create a portrait of the patients whom you serve. As markets "mature" with respect to managed care, there is an increase in the shifting of the risk for paying for medical services from the MCOs to the providers. Just as the insurance companies build databases of information in order to manage the risks they undertake, so must medical practices build and analyze the data available to them with respect to the utilization of services by their patients.

Unfortunately, physicians generally do not have access to sound data regarding utilization of physician services. The Health Insurance Association of America (HIAA) does compile utilization data based upon commercial insurance claims. These data are available to insurers, and are now available to providers, but the cost can easily be thousands of dollars. The challenge facing a practice that is taking on risk is to forecast the utilization of services for which it will be financially as well as operationally responsible.

A practice can hire an actuary to work with it to develop utilization projections. This may be an expensive undertaking, however, as the practice assumes more risk, it may prove to be an investment well worth the expense.

Nevertheless, in preparation for assuming more risk, the practice can compile its own database looking at its experience with its current patients. From this data, you can analyze the rate of utilization by service and look for any variances among geographic areas, or by payer.

Many businesses overlook the wealth of information that lies within their information systems. One of the keys to success is the ability to "mine" your databases, locating and extracting data and information that aids decision making. In the following pages, I will suggest some steps to take in that direction.

The first step would be for the practice to look at its own patient data and produce the following report. For each zip code, present the following data (Table 1-1):

TABLE 1–1

Utilization by Age and Sex

Age	# Male	(%)	# Female	(%)	Total	(%)
0–17						
18–44						
45–64						
65+						
Total						

TABLE 1–2

Utilization Rate by Age and Sex: Service A

Age	# Services	Rate/1,000 Patients	Est. # HMO Lives	Projected Services
0–17				
18–44				
45–64				
65+				
Total				

Note: Determine number of active patients (any patient seen in past two years)

It also would be valuable to run the same data report for each major service, although not necessarily for each zip code unless there is a sufficient number of patients. The major services would be:

- Office visits.
- Office consultations.
- Hospital visits.
- Hospital consultations.
- Procedures (with breakdowns for the more prevalent or revenue-generating procedures).

Absent other information, your current experience is the best predictor of the future. As managed care takes hold, the growth in utilization will probably slow and reverse itself. The underlying assumption here is that the *rate* of utilization of services for the HMO population you will be assuming risk for is similar to or the same as the rate of utilization of your current patient population, adjusted for age and sex (Table 1-2).

This chart should be repeated for each major service. Once you have established the rate of utilization of each service, you can then apply that rate per thousand patients to the estimated number of patients—then known as covered lives—that the HMO will be sending to you for care.

TABLE 1–3

Current Patient Population by Payer, Age, Sex

HMO # 1

Age	# Male	(%)	# Female	(%)	Total	(%)
0–17						
18–44						
45–64						
65+						
Total						

This analysis works best for primary care practices, since HMOs assign a defined, identifiable group of patients to a practice. For specialty practices, however, patients enter the practice for treatment and then "leave"—patients of specialty practices are "active" patients by definition. Specialty practices may find that it makes more sense to look at the cost of service per patient on a per patient per month (PPPM) basis. In Chapter 4, dealing with capitation, I will present in further detail the ways in which to assess capitation rates.

The specifics of which procedures to look for will vary from practice to practice and specialty to specialty.

Table 1-3 presents fundamental data concerning a practice's patient base: the distribution by age and sex. It is helpful to sort this data on each of the following bases:

- Total practice.
- MCO patients as a group.
  - As a subset, look at each MCO separately.
- Commercial, non-MCO patients.
- Medicare patients.
- Medicaid patients.

The goal of building these reports is to then compare utilization among the different payer groups. Within the MCO market, it would be valuable to see if there are differences in utilization, which could be driven by the demographics of the patient population or it could be driven by the utilization management controls imposed by the health plan. This information is just part of the tools a practice has to develop a portrait of their "customers" and as aid in negotiating rates and contracts.

Repeat this report for each HMO for which you have a contract. The age groups suggested here are common breaks in utilization trends. If your practice handles pediatrics, you will also want to break out the "under one-year-old" population, as this group is a high user of services due to routine well baby care as well as illness, parent inexperience, and the difficulty in diagnosing and assessing routine problems (the patients don't speak).

The next set of information to collect is financial:

- Determine total charges by service for each quarter over the past three years.
- Determine total collections by service for each calendar quarter over the past three years.
- Compute the charges and collections on a PPPM basis, using the number of unique patients in the practice as the denominator.

Lastly, I would look at this data in several ways:

- For each quarter for each of the past three years, look for variations by year.
- Look for variations by quarter—your practice may experience seasonal variations.

Compiling all this information gives you a set of critical data that you will need in order to rapidly address proposed contracts from managed care plans, particularly when presented with a capitated or other risk-sharing arrangement. In later chapters, you will see how this information is put to use.

Through all the changes, all the new players, there is one constant: the people who pay the premiums, the employers. And that is what all the turmoil in healthcare is about—the employers. What we are all scrambling over is our piece of the premium dollar—and it's a shrinking dollar at that. Employers are employing increasingly sophisticated tools in their effort to decide who gets their business—the right to care for their employees. Increasingly, MCOs and employers are limiting the group of providers who will be receiving business. For providers, then, instead of having, say, 1,000,000 potential individual customers in a market of 1,000,000 people, there may be 50 or 100 customers—MCOs and employers who are self-insured or contract directly. And that number may decrease also as the MCO industry shakes out and consolidates and employers band together in buying consortiums to make the selection decisions. For medical practices, then, their challenge is to find a niche and wend their way through the myriad of new competitors snapping at their turf and to capture their piece of the premium dollar. In the chapters ahead, we'll discuss the strategies and techniques for doing just that.

2 CHAPTER

Analyzing the MCO Contract

Your first contact with a managed care plan may come in the form of a thick envelope that lands on your desk one day. These envelopes are about the size of those you anxiously awaited from the college of your choice when you were a high school senior. In the package often will be brochures, a copy of a contract with a letter saying "this is who we are, here's a contract, sign here." Don't sign. If you gain nothing else from this book learn this:

Rule #1: Read the contract

I make such a big point about it here and in my seminars only because you would be amazed at how many practices have come to me with a problem they are having with a managed care organization (MCO). The first words out of my mouth are, "What does the contract say?" and their response is a blank look, a sheepish downward gazing of the eyes, and a quiet acknowledgment that they have never read the contract. Worse yet are physicians who sign contracts and never share the contract with their staff.

Rule #2: Share the contract

Unlike your traditional relationship with a standard indemnity plan, with a managed care organization, you the physician and other providers have a contractual agreement with the health plan. This document is a legally enforceable agreement—let me repeat—*legally enforceable.* This means that your ultimate remedy is a court of law. This changes the nature of the relationship dramatically. When you bill an indemnity carrier, you are billing as a courtesy to the patient. With a managed care contract you are billing for your services directly to the party who has a contractual responsibility to pay you, not the patient. With indemnity plans you have the option to go directly to the patient for payment if you do not have a response or payment from the carrier within 30 to 60 days. Under a managed care arrangement, that option is usually not present. You can request assistance from the patient in collecting from the MCO, but ultimately you, and you alone, are responsible for pursuing and collecting your own bills.

CONTRACT STRUCTURE

Legal contracts have a common thread in their structure and content, and contracts with managed care organizations are no different. In this chapter, we will approach the contract review from several perspectives, including:

- Legal requirements.
- The impact on your practice from three perspectives—finances, clinical practices, and internal operations.
- Background information in preparation for negotiating a contract.

For the legal requirements, the reader must retain the assistance of a competent attorney in his locality. State laws vary from state to state, so you need someone who understands the particular laws of your state. Just as the construction of a will must be written in a certain way in order to achieve your personal goals for your estate, so must you make sure that the language you negotiate in a managed care plan achieves what you want it to achieve.

In selecting an attorney to assist you, look for one who has at least some experience dealing with these contracts. The attorney who handles your retirement plan is not necessarily the person who should handle managed care contracts. The hospital's attorney also is not a great choice, as there is a very real potential for a conflict of interest situation. There are a number of attorneys who have experience with these contracts. It is also possible to use an attorney in a distant city, since there is often little need for face-to-face interaction. Most, if not all, of the advisory services will be rendered by phone and fax (or, nowadays, e-mail). It doesn't make a lot of difference whether you are calling from down the street or 1,000 miles away.

To locate an attorney, references from colleagues are one route. Your accountant is another, as is the hospital's attorney. The state medical society sometimes maintains lists, as does your malpractice carrier. The National Health Lawyers Association is a leading professional society, and it maintains a listing of members.

Even with a recommendation, do your homework. You would like to develop an ongoing relationship with one attorney whom you will be able to rely on and call upon when needed. Ask for references, and call those references. When making a reference check, your questions might include:

- What kind of work did Mr. Attorney do for you? (A general idea, without confidential details.)
- Did you feel that you received the attention you needed?
- Were your questions answered so that you could understand them? Did he explain the business and / or legal rationale behind the advice given so that you could make a better business decision?
- Were phone calls returned in a timely manner? How long for a typical call?
- How did she treat your staff when calling you or otherwise working with your staff?
- Were costs and expenses within reason?

Legal Perspective

The notion of a contract is that both parties are entering into an agreement where there is an exchange; one party will be doing something in return for something of value being conveyed by the other party. An employment contract is an agreement where a person agrees to work for an employer for a defined period of time, in return for being given a certain position with certain authority and responsibilities and being paid a salary and other benefits for that entire time period. The agreement need not be fair or equitable in order to be enforceable in a court of law, but it must conform to certain guidelines. In addition, a court will not enforce the terms of a contract that either calls for an illegal act to be performed, creates an illegal situation (price fixing is an example), or is contrary to public policy.

Impact on Operations

In analyzing the contract, there are three operational perspectives from which to view the contract: financial, clinical practices, and internal operations.

1. Financial perspective. Analyzing the contract from a financial perspective comes down to a very simple set of questions:
   a. How will we be paid?
   b. How much will we be paid?
   c. What will we be paid for? What will we not be paid for?
   d. When and how often will we be paid?
2. Clinical practices perspective. This is becoming the greatest area of concern. All too many MCOs are interposing themselves into the patient treatment process, and are virtually dictating what treatments will be provided, where it will be provided, and when. Some plans have enacted "gag" rules, restricting what physicians say to patients about treatments that are not being suggested or authorized by the MCO, while others have drug formularies that restrict the payment for newer, more expensive drugs. Other MCOs simply restrict the universe from which patients can obtain care.

3. Operations perspective. There are a number of requirements in the typical MCO contract that will require procedural changes within the practice. What is most troublesome is not the need to track, say, referral forms, but the fact that each health plan has differing sets of providers in its network, and within a single health plan there may be dozens of different networks.

ANALYZING THE CONTRACT

As you begin your analysis of the contract, there are seven key points that you will want to focus on: (1) preliminaries and recitations; (2) compensation/pricing; (3) covered services/restrictions; (4) stop loss; (5) utilization management practices/treatment quidelines; (6) term/termination and renewal provisions; and (7) indemnification. We will discuss each of these in turn.

Preliminaries and Recitations

These are the opening sections of a contract that state the names of the parties entering into the contract and the purpose for entering into the contract. In some contracts there may some "where as" clauses that outline the reasons for entering into the contract. In analyzing the contract, you are looking to see that the names of the two parties are correct, the type of legal organization (corporation, partnership, etc.), and in which state the organization is formed. Do note the legal name and "doing business as" (DBA) name of the MCO. A DBA name is a name or trademark that a business uses in dealing with its customers. For example, many franchise stores may be organized by the franchise owner as "Joe and Mary's Restaurant Corp.," but they do business as a McDonald's restaurant. For their purposes, their DBA is McDonald's. For legal, liability, and other business reasons, a health plan may have a name it uses nationally, but it may have a separate corporation organized in each state or market in which it operates. Sometimes, the local corporation may be a joint venture involving a local group, hospital, or other investors. The importance here is that you understand clearly with whom you are signing a contract and entering into a business relationship.

Compensation/Pricing

This is the heart of the contract and the issue that will involve the most negotiation. If the contract is a capitated one, the pricing is simply listed as the per member per month (PMPM). Under a negotiated fee schedule you need to carefully examine the fee schedule. Some plans have been known to offer contracts without offering the fee schedule. One notorious plan in upstate New York will tell physicians that they will be paid approximately 137 percent of the Medicare rate, but they will never formally acknowledge the rate. In some of these situations the plan may tell you that it cannot possibly provide the full fee schedule, because the full fee schedule would entail all 10,000 or so common procedure terminology (CPT) codes. Secondly, the plan does not want its full fee schedule floating around town, which is likely to happen if it starts sending it out. The plan will ask you, and it is reasonable to respond, to provide it with a list of your CPT codes for which you need to know the fee. You should be able to generate this promptly from your computer system. Some plans, unfortunately, will demand that you provide them with a copy of your fee schedule, or even the schedules from other plans. This is proprietary information. If the plan persists, one approach would be to provide a proposed fee schedule, marked as "proposed fee schedule" or simply "fee schedule" which may in fact be higher than your standard private fees. This schedule will give you a basis for negotiating from then on.

Covered Services/Restrictions

This section is important in all contracts, but it is of particular and critical importance in a capitated contract.

In all MCO contracts, there will be some restrictions on where and when referrals can be made for any nonprimary care service. It is one thing to know that the universe within which you can refer patients is limited. It is quite another to be told that the MCO will not pay for a service that the physician believes to be in the best interest of the patient. Not only that, some MCOs will try to prohibit physicians from discussing treatment options at all with their patients if the discussion will lead into areas that the MCO will not be covering. These so-called gag rules are under increasing attack, and they are being outlawed in some states and even voluntarily dropped by some MCOs.

In a capitated contract, you have agreed with the other party, the health plan, to provide certain services for a group of covered lives as they need the services, whenever they need the services. In return, you are to be paid a certain amount of money—the capitation fee (or rate)—for each member for each month, regardless of the number of services that you provide in the month.

Again, different from indemnity plans, which will pay for any valid, medically necessary service you render, managed care plans may in fact define the scope of the services for which the plan will pay you. This is of particular importance when it comes to a capitation arrangement, in which you are being paid PMPM to provide a defined scope of services for the patient. The critical word here is "defined." As a primary care physician, your interest is in knowing and understanding the scope of services that you are expected to provide under the capitation rate and what services you might be able to provide that would not be covered by the cap rate and would be paid for on a fee-for-service or other basis. Secondly, a family practitioner who does obstetrics would be very interested in knowing whether she would be allowed to continue to perform deliveries and how they would be paid for or whether the health plan would prohibit her doing so for the plan's members. The specialist has a similar situation. If capitated, what services will the specialist be responsible for and which ones can he expect to be provided by the primary care physician? One of the goals of a managed care arrangement is to push down services to the least expensive setting and least expensive provider, in this situation, to get away from the specialists and let the primary care physicians handle the situation. An example of this is an uncomplicated myocardial infarction (MI). A general surgeon may have training in certain subspecialty areas in which she performs work but needs to understand whether the plan will allow her to continue to do the subspecialty work. Conversely, a surgeon who is principally a subspecialist may do some general surgery and needs to understand whether the plan will allow him to continue to do so.

Stop Loss

As discussed earlier under capitation arrangement, there is the potential that a very bad case will expend significantly more time and cost to a practice than is anticipated under the PMPM being paid. In assuming the risk for the services to be provided in return for a fixed fee, the practice has made certain assumptions as to the volume and intensity of services that will be provided. People being people, some patients will unfortunately require very expensive care, expenses that far exceed the projections. To limit this exposure, practices can purchase stop loss insurance. As the name implies, it "stops" the "losses"—losses being the expenses in provided services under the health plan contract. Stop loss insurance can be purchased from a private carrier, or through the HMO. The contract needs to be read carefully to determine whether there is a notation and money set aside within the agreement for a stop-loss arrangement. In some instances the contract will specify a dollar amount for services rendered above which the practice will receive additional payment and a percentage of a negotiated fee or discounted fee arrangement. It also may specify where the services are rendered and set different dollar amounts if the service is rendered in hospital or out of hospital. These sections must be read very carefully and clearly understood.

Utilization Management Practices/Treatment Guidelines

A few years ago there was a run of scandals involving utilization management by certain health plans. The scandals seem to have died down, but it is important that you understand who exactly is providing your utilization management (UM) services for the plan. Some plans have made it a business unit to provide these administrative services to other health plans. All of this is fine; you just want to know who is providing the UM services and which set of standards they are using. In many states, UM providers are licensed by the state insurance department.

The plan may require you to follow certain guidelines in treating certain presented situations. A primary example of this is in psychiatry, where the plan's UM guidelines may require the use of older drugs as opposed to some newer drugs, in conjunction with psychotherapy. The plans may restrict if not severely limit the use of psychotherapy in treating certain psychiatric situations. Use of antibiotics is another example, and certain other expensive therapies may require certain kinds of workups and diagnostic criteria before these treatments are approved. You need to be aware of what may impact you. If you are having problems being paid with indemnity carriers now, for example, questions are being asked and paper documentation is requested on a routine basis, then assume you will have the same problem with a managed care organization. In these situations, raise the question up front in your contract negotiations with the managed care plan as to how it treats these situations. This kind of preventative action will solve a lot of problems down the road.

Term/Termination and Renewal Provisions

Since a contract defines a business relationship and the nature of the exchange, contracts will include a section that will address the length of time the relationship will exist under the terms of the agreement. While both parties can agree to renegotiate the terms at any time, placing a time limit on the agreement compels both parties to discuss the terms for continuing the relationship. If a new agreement is not reached, even if the terms do not change, the contract expires at the end of the term and the relationship is severed.

There are several concepts that are central to the term and termination:

- Termination.
- Notice.
- With cause / without cause.
- Mutual termination rights.

It is not unusual for an MCO contract to come through to you with a provision that allows the MCO to *terminate* the contract *without cause*—meaning without giving a reason. However, the *notice* of the intention to terminate the contract must be provided to you in writing at least a specified number of days (30 or 60 days would be common) in advance of the date that the termination would become effective. You may not however, have the same right. You often will have to bring up this disparity in the contract negotiation, that you were not given the same right—*mutual termination*—as the MCO in the first proposed contract. Usually, this is a simple matter to dispense with and the MCO will agree to the mutual termination clause. Be very careful to insist that all such notices be delivered by certified mail, return receipt requested. This method is a proof of mailing and of delivery, and such delivery is mandatory for changing critical parts of the contract (such as, say, whether you even have a contract).

In the case of MCO contracts, the MCO needs to insure that it has sufficient provider capacity to serve its members. For that reason, it cannot be placed in a situation where a provider terminates its contract unless the MCO has time to replace that provider's capacity. In the case of a small provider, as are most medical practices, the patients probably can be distributed among the existing provider capacity. In these situations, a relatively short notice period of 30 or 60 days (60 days is preferable from your perspective) would be sufficient. A hospital, on the other hand, is quite another story. A notice for a hospital can be six or more months, for the simple reason that the loss of hospital capacity or the hospital's geographic coverage will not be easy to replace.

Any contract can of course be broken, regardless of the term. It is only a question of whether and how much the damages are that will be paid. Managed care contracts typically are written with a one year term. As MCOs mature and markets begin to stabilize, we are seeing increasing numbers of multiyear contracts.

Renewal provisions also can come in several ways. A contract may provide that the contract will renew automatically unless written notification is made 30, 60, or 90 days in advance to the other party that the contract will not be renewed. These are referred to as "evergreen" contracts. Some contracts have a defined limit of one year or more, but they must be renewed beginning at a defined period of time, perhaps 60 days in advance. Others have a simple defined term and, unless renewed by both parties signing a new agreement (which may simply be a letter extending the terms with any changes noted), the contract expires at the termination date.

Indemnification

This is one of my favorite sections of a contract. Again, be forewarned—the first contract proposed by the MCO may come through with a provision whereby you will "hold harmless, indemnify, and defend " the MCO for any legal or regulatory actions arising out of the care of patients. What such language does is shift all of the risk and financial responsibility for any action a patient may take against you or the plan squarely to you. You may then be defending and will be financially responsible for any damages, even if the cause was an action by the MCO.

Let me make this clear—such a provision is never, ever to be signed by you. These clauses are not unusual in proposed contracts. You, however, cannot and should not take on responsibility for insuring someone else. Your position is that you will be responsible for what you do, and the MCO can be responsible for what it does. Your insurance carriers—professional liability and general liability—usually will not be willing to add other parties to your policy. The language of the contract must be changed to remove the indemnification clause, and replace it with language that accomplishes the following:

- Each party to the contract is responsible for its own actions, and any legal costs or liabilities that arise.
- Both parties agree to cooperate with each other in the defenses of an action brought against one or the other, or both. (Remember: your interests may not be the same as the interests of the health plan, so a joint defense may not be your best course of action.)

The contract may require that you maintain a certain level of professional liability insurance, which probably is not very different from that which is required by hospitals for medical staff privileges. You should contact your professional liability carrier to make sure that your coverage is sufficient and that the MCO contract language is not posing any significant issues for you.

Since the MCO brought it up, physicians are well advised to ask the MCO about its liability coverage. It would not be unusual for an MCO to be self-insured for a significant amount of risk before its policies take hold. If the MCO's coverage is not sufficient, however, you do not want to be in the position of finding that a court judgment defaults to you as the defendant with the adequate coverage.

DUE DILIGENCE CHECKLIST

It's all in the preparation.

Preparing to negotiate a contract with an MCO may be *the* critical task, almost as important as the negotiation itself. This period of preparation is a learning process that involves gathering and analyzing facts, information, impressions, judgments, and rumors. This period also can be characterized as a "due diligence" process, sharing the term used in the period between the signing of a contract and the closing when purchasing a house or a business. In conducting the due diligence for a managed care contract, there are two goals, one short term, and one long term:

- Short term: preparation for negotiating the contract.
- Long term: preparation for implementation of the contract.

Many practices have found that using a checklist to review managed care contracts is an effective and efficient way of making sure that you have collected all the information you need and checked the different sections of the contract so that you understand the implications of the document completely. You want to know who you are doing business with and understand the implications of signing and entering into a business arrangement with them.

On the following pages we will walk through a checklist approach as a guide to evaluating contracts.

1. Name of the Organization

You are now preparing to enter into a contractual relationship with this company, so you must know exactly who the other party is. Many plans are subsidiaries of larger organizations or may be managed by a different organization, depending upon the locale and state in which they are operating.

2. History

History tells a lot about an organization—where it came from, its ethics, performance, and reputation. You want to know when and where the organization was founded, how long it has been in existence, and whether there have been mergers or takeovers in its history. This is also an opportune time to identify any significant past legal problems.

3. What Type of Relationship Is This?

Is this an HMO, PPO, Independent Practice Association (IPA), network, direct contract, or some other kind of arrangement? This is also a check point to insure that this is not a silent PPO arrangement.

4. Ownership/Form of Organization

The MCO may be a subsidiary of a larger organization, part of a joint venture (say, with a competitor or predator), or simply an old fashioned scam. I can't emphasize the point enough—you must know and understand with whom you're doing business. By asking questions, you will identify:

- The corporate name and DBA (doing business as) name used in your state.
- The name of any parent organization(s) (there may be several layers of subsidiaries).
- Any joint venture partners or significant investors, particularly if such investors are from your local market.

If the MCO is a publicly traded company, there is a great deal of information that will be available. Publicly traded companies are required to file numerous reports that are available for little or no charge (particularly if you have Internet access). Public companies also are the subject of analyses and investor research reports and are followed by the business news media; these products often are available as well.

Your first stop is with the company itself to obtain what many call an investor's packet. An investor's packet typically will include the company's annual report, Form 10-K, quarterly reports, and perhaps press releases. Public companies usually will provide these documents in the investor's packet format or individually upon request to anyone who calls. Callers usually are going to be investors or potential investors, so obtaining these documents is easy.

If you have Internet access, those documents that are filed with the Securities and Exchange Commission (SEC) are available through the EDGAR system in the SEC's web site. (You can access these documents at the SEC web site address: *www.SEC.com*. Then, simply follow the directions to search the EDGAR system. You will need to know the name of the company. All of the filings are now made electronically and can be downloaded.)

With the explosion of Internet use, many companies have their own web sites. United Healthcare, U.S. Healthcare, some of the Blue Cross plans, and some state health departments all have web sites that are worth exploring and checking in on from time to time.

The key document you are looking for is the SEC annual filing known as Form 10-K. Many are familiar with the annual report, which has pretty pictures, glowing statements from the company CEO, and the soaring prose of "vision statements." A Form 10-K, on the other hand, has no pictures, it is presented in fairly plain type, and there is a certain amount of required information that needs to be in the document. What is important to you are the sections dealing with business strategy. Companies, you must understand, have a great deal of latitude in how they respond to these questions, but some companies are much more forthcoming. As an example, HealthSource, a New Hampshire-based HMO company, outlines its strategy as:

- Its desire to partner with physicians as the best means to achieving cost control.
- Its desire to enter into joint ventures (and it names some joint venture partners).
- Its preference for smaller markets.

The HealthSource Form 10-K also lists the board of directors and includes a three- or four-line biography. In reading the HealthSource Form 10-K, you will see that all the members of the board are physicians, many of whom are still in active practice.

From this, you now have several pieces of information that may be helpful in negotiating a contract:

1. The names of joint venture partners who can be contacted for references.
2. The stated belief that "physicians are the key to controlling costs" and the preference for "partnering with physicians" is language that you can use in the negotiation—you would be "reflecting" to their representative the sharing of their business principals.

5. Corporate and Local Officers/Management

As it is said, "All healthcare is local" and "Business is really about people." These hold true with MCO contracts as well. Although the contract bears the names of companies, it is the people on both sides who will make the contract work well, or work poorly. In this step, you will identify the key officers on a corporate level and on a regional or local level. The positions that you will be most interested in include:

- Corporate CEO.
- Corporate marketing director.
- Corporate director of provider relations.
- Corporate medical director.
- Regional chief executive / director.
- Regional medical director.
- Regional marketing director.
- Regional provider relations director.
- Claims management director.

Where to get this information? Asking directly sometimes works, but don't be surprised if the MCO representative clams up and plays dumb. All too often, "customer service" is an alien concept to MCOs. There are several sources out there. The American Association of Health Plans, out of the Washington, D.C. area, and the private firm Interstudy of St. Paul, Minnesota, both publish directories that list all HMOs and include listings of key corporate officers. (See Appendix G for contact information.)

As a practical matter, the most important names to you are going to be the regional and local people, for they are the ones who will be managing your contract.

6. A Copy of the Agreement, Fee Schedule, and All Referenced Attachments and Exhibits

You think this is funny? You're reading this and thinking, "This is so obvious—why do I need to check this off?"

Well, guess what. Ask around. It will amaze, astonish, and horrify you the number of very smart people who never read the contract. Or, they don't bother to get all the attachments; the contract will refer to policies and procedures that the signing provider never sees or reads. Worse yet, there are occasional instances where HMOs have tried to get providers to sign a letter agreeing to the terms of a contract that "will follow later." And smart people actually sign these things!

There is nothing to discuss without a full copy of the agreement, with all blanks filled in or noted as "not applicable," and all policies and procedures that are referenced in the contract (such as a grievance procedure) included.

Another horror—smart people signing contracts without (1) seeing the fee schedule, and (2) understanding how and when they will be paid.

Although there is much to discuss in a contract negotiation without the fee schedule, the fees are the central issue. You may be willing to trade off on a number of issues in return for an improved fee schedule.

Some MCOs will provide the fee schedule when they first make contact with you. Since this first contact may be by mail, it is not unreasonable that they will not send a proposed fee schedule through the mail to a party who is essentially unknown to them and risk having their fee schedule end up all over town.

When first requesting the fee schedule, present it as a matter-of-fact request—you do not want this request to be treated as the first move in a negotiation. In making the request, you will need to define the scope of the fees that you need. Again, MCOs operate in a very competitive market, so they are not about to release their entire fee schedule and risk having copies fall into the hands of their competition. You may be asked to provide a list of the common procedure terminology (CPT) codes that you bill for. As a practical matter, practices (other than large multispecialty groupings of some sort) use only a limited portion of the CPT codes. Your computer system should be able to produce a list of all the codes that you have billed for in the past year. The MCO can then return to you a list of proposed fees.

7. Services to be Provided

The first issue here is to insure that you will be allowed to provide those services that are part of your practice. A family practitioner, for instance, may do obstetrics in his practice. But he may find that the MCO will not allow him to offer that service for its patients. Or, you may be a family practitioner who does not provide obstetrics but the MCO may want you to, or the contract may come through that way. In either case, this is one of the critical sections of the contract because it defines your responsibility to the MCO and its patients. You must be prepared to provide the services stated in the contract.

This section may also include language that requires a physician to be available 24 hours a day, seven days a week. For most practices, this is not a problem in and of itself—round the clock coverage is taken care of either through the group or through sharing cover with other physicians in the community. Problems may arise, however, if all of the physicians who cover patients are not members of the same health plans. This usually is not a problem within a group practice, although there are groups where all of the physicians are not members of the same health plans.

Some health plans will pay covering physicians when they serve a plan member. Others may require the contracting physician to make their own financial arrangements with the covering physicians. When a contract is being signed, ask the health plan how they will pay your covering physicians, or be prepared to work out an arrangement among the physicians as to how MCO patients will be handled for payment purposes—including the option of paying the other physicians out of your capitation fees.

8. Review of the Scope of Benefits in Offered Plans

The services covered under MCO plans are usually more generous than those covered under traditional indemnity plans. In this step, you will be requesting copies of summaries (if not the full documents) for the various plans offered by the MCO. The goal of this review is to:

- Insure that the services that you provide are covered.
- Identify any limitations that affect your services.
- Identify any differences in the patient's financial obligations that effect your services.

Mental health is one major specialty that has traditionally faced serious restrictions in the scope of benefits for patients. It is not unusual for an MCO mental health benefit to have a $50 co-payment, versus $10–15 for other physician services, and a yearly dollar cap for expenses and a lifetime cap of $25–50,000, which is significantly lower than a more common lifetime maximum expenditure of $1,000,000.

9. Geographic Coverage/Membership/Demographics of Covered Lives

The only real reason for signing an MCO contract is to gain the market share and patient volume from the patients the MCO can bring to the table—their members, or "covered lives." You will be collecting information as to the geographic area where the MCO is currently licensed to operate as well as areas where the MCO plans to expand (or, I should note, where you can deduce that they will eventually move into).

Ask for the current membership data for the MCO. Ideally, you would like this information not only for your entire market area, but for the "submarket" area that you can realistically serve (e.g., geographic area, certain zip codes, etc.).

The other important piece of information is the "disenrollment rate." The disenrollment rate is that percentage of members who disenroll or leave the plan for any number of reasons. This could include an employer dropping the plan as a provider, which is a source of information in and of itself. In addition, members may deselect and choose other health coverage due to dissatisfaction with the plan's operations or perhaps how care is rendered. You should know that this disenrollment rate typically is public information, in the event that the plan resists providing this data. If the plan is new to your market area, you can ask for this information for other areas, particularly market areas similar to yours. This gives you some indication of how the plan does in other markets. Obviously, be aware that plans do differ in how they operate from market to market. The well respected plans may in fact have a "wayward" plan within their organization. Health plans are also being asked to report the physician disenrollment rate, which the plan should make available to you.

In MCO contracts where you have taken on some risk, such as withhold/risk pool and capitation arrangements, one of the key issues you face is projecting the utilization of your services. In order to do that, you will need to know the demographic distribution of the covered lives for whom you will be responsible. The data need to be presented by zip code, showing the distribution of lives by sex and age. (More on this in Chapter 4.)

Demographic data are collected by the MCO and, in many cases, such as with HMOs, there are filings with the state insurance department that will contain this information. Be forewarned that all MCOs may not be forthcoming with this data, and you may have to be forceful in seeking it. Be forceful.

10. Current Provider Network

If the MCO already is operating in your market, there should be no problems obtaining the list of other providers. If it is new to your area, you may want to look at the provider list from other markets, particularly those similarly sized.

The provider lists are important to you so that you can identify the providers with whom you currently do business and those areas where you may have to change your relationships. Every practice has a small circle of providers with whom it has ongoing relationships—the specialists it refers patients to, where its lab work is done, and which hospitals it uses for admissions and outpatient work. MCOs define their own universe of providers, and you must stay within this universe when making referral decisions.

Some providers require that you formalize your relationship with them. Hospitals require admission to their medical staff, and some facilities may require that transfer agreements and certain protocols be followed. If you are a specialist of any sort (i.e., receiving referrals from primary care physicians), you must initiate a relationship with these physicians and their office staffs who don't know who you are, what you can do, and how well you do it. Do remember that even MCO plans provide patients with a choice of specialists. The universe of choices may be limited and defined, but there are choices. You will need to develop these relationships in order to insure that you get the referrals you need. (See Chapter 9 on marketing.)

11. Major Employer Groups

Just as you will be assigned patients in bulk by an MCO, an MCO writes policies for groups of lives that can vary widely in size. Major, large employers are more likely to be self-insured and using the MCO as a claims administrator. So if an employer decides to move its business to another plan, the MCO loses the business, which means that that group of covered lives—employees plus dependents—moves with it. For example, AT&T moved 40,000 employees plus dependents—a total of 100,000 people—into one plan administered by U.S. Healthcare (merging with Aetna at this writing).

The importance of the employer list is that it serves as a source of references for the MCO. Plans typically will be very proud of a high profile, well-respected company that has selected them. In marketing terms, these company clients are known as the "influencers." Influencers are those who, because of their respect in the marketplace, lead others to purchase a similar product. A plan with a high-profile employer client list is more likely to be a successful plan.

Finally, you are interested in seeing whether your patients are covered by the employers being signed up or targeted by the plan. One of the pieces of information you should be collecting for your patients is who their employer is, from both spouses, regardless of who the primary insurance carrier is. As the plan is signing up new employer groups, this will help you identify how many of your patients will be eligible to join.

12. Conduct a Reference Check on the MCO

Why not? The MCO has done some homework on you, why shouldn't you do a background check on it? If the plan is operating in your market, call locally, and if it is new to your area, call references in the markets where it already operates. For most smaller practices, it might be considered presumptuous to ask the MCO for references. Nothing stops you, however, from calling on practices similar to yours to ask how the MCO performs. To locate individuals to call, use the membership directories of your professional societies such as the Medical Group Management Association (MGMA).

For a sample of questions to ask in your reference check, see Appendix B.

13. Discuss the MCO's Marketing Plan

One of the principal reasons a practice accepts a lower fee schedule or a risk sharing agreement with an MCO is the promise that the health plan will bring patients to the practice—helping to keep current patients as well as directing new patients to the practice. Therefore, you will want to initiate a discussion with the MCO representatives regarding:

- Growth in the past year.
- Growth targets for the coming year.
- New benefit plans being developed.
- New marketing initiatives.
- Plans for geographic expansion.
- Assessment of competition.

You can help move such a conversation along by volunteering your own information about competitors' actions and your own assessments. Proprietary information with which you've been entrusted is, of course, off limits, but a lot of business interactions are "eased" through this exchange of information. People like to talk about their businesses and their industry—use this mutual interest to help you gather and trade competitive information.

14. Opportunities for "Designated Provider" Status

This doesn't refer to PPOs. If your practice offers a specialized or otherwise unique service, you are looking to gather all of the MCO's business; your practice is designated by the MCO as the only (or one of a select few) site where a certain service can be provided for the MCO's members. In return for the volume, you of course can then offer a lower price. Specialized testing, particularly when there is expensive equipment whose cost is being amortized, is an ideal candidate for such an arrangement.

Designated provider arrangements also can be established on a geographic basis. As an example, your practice would contract to provide all allergy testing for the southeastern sections of the market area. Any member whose residence is within a set of zip codes (or some other definition of geography, although zip codes are easy and objective) would have to be referred to your practice if the primary care physician were making such a referral. In these situations, the MCO system of restricted provider networks is magically transformed into a wonderful business and clinical tool. It all depends upon your viewpoint.

15. The Claim Billing System

Although this should be a simple matter, it is critical that these questions be asked and verified. While most MCOs use the standard forms and systems for claims, there are a few who decide to be heroes and invent their own. Here are the points to check:

- Is the HCFA 1500 form or format used for claims filing?
- Is the standard American Medical Association (AMA) CPT-4 coding used?
- Is the National HCPCS coding used?
- Are other supplementary codes used?

- Is electronic billing available? Ask about technical requirements and get your practice management software vendor involved immediately.
- Is electronic remittance available? Again, ask about any technical requirements and get your vendor involved. The issue here simply may be how the remittance advice is transmitted to you. The funds transfer will be handled by the banks involved through the Federal Reserve system.
- What is the payment cycle? Are there guarantees for the processing of claims and remittance of funds? Are there any penalties if claims processing is delayed?

MCO contracts generally will require claims to be filed, even in the presence of a capitation methodology. Even if the carrier does not require claim filing, it is critical that you continue to code properly and completely and record all of the services and charges in your computer system. You need the history as documentation to support rate increases, as a basis for managing your practice, and in the event patients move to other carriers; you will then have a complete history to forecast utilization and costs.

16. Provider Representatives for Claims Management Issues and General Contract Issues

Given the complexities of the rules surrounding MCO plans and the inherent nature of filing claims with insurance carriers, there will be claims management problems and issues to resolve with the MCO. There is little reason why almost all of the problems can't be resolved easily with a phone call.

Ask if the MCO assigns a designated person from provider relations to act as your principal contact with the plan. If it doesn't assign one person, you will need to know the name of the director of provider relations, for there are some issues that will need attention from management.

Claims management—the people who receive, process, and pay your claims—is one group within the MCO with whom you will have frequent contact during your relationship with the MCO. As a matter of course, most inquiries will go through normal channels. Some plans, however, assign individuals to specific providers. Your interest here is to identify who that person is. After the contract is signed, you can call that person and begin to establish a relationship.

17. Primary Care Physician Approvals Required

Are there services that may not require that the primary care physician (PCP) initiate the referral? More importantly, are there any financial implications to the PCP for services that he did not have to approve? For specialists, the issue is slightly different: namely, are there services that they may want to order after the initial workup and consult on a patient? If so, will they need to obtain PCP approval before proceeding, or will the specialist have some latitude as to what he can authorize? Absent a risk-sharing agreement, specialists usually will have to get PCP clearance.

Some services may require approval by the plan's medical director as well. Services requiring this level of approval will tend to be certain tertiary level services, services that are only available "out of plan" or otherwise not fall neatly within the benefit description of the specific policies and plans being marketed. For example, I dealt with an HMO that required the regional medical director to approve all left heart catheterizations, a procedure that is relatively straight-forward, low risk, and with little history of abuse.

So ask. As a rule, any service that has faced medical necessity reviews, uses high technology equipment located within your practice, or has gained notoriety as an overused service (cesarean sections are the classic example) is likely to face more scrutiny from the MCO's claims management group. As part of your due diligence, you will raise the issue of the services, including:

- How to bill for the service (e.g., coding and any documentation to be submitted with the claim).
- Any specific documentation the MCO wants either to be submitted with the claim or available for audit.
- Whether the PCP authorization will be sufficient, whether the plan will need to precertify the service, and/or whether the medical director or other level will need to issue approval.

The "preventative medicine" rule applies here, so take the medicine. You'll feel better.

18. Procedures for Out-of-Plan Approval

As discussed in Item (17), if you may have to send patients out of the area or out of the plan for a specific service, raise the issue now and meet with the medical director. Your goal in the meeting is to outline: (1) the circumstances when certain patients need to be sent out of plan, because only certain institutions can provide the service; (2) the protocol(s) you use in making the determination to make such a referral; and (3) the expected benefit to the patient. By initiating the discussion and discussing your protocols with the medical director, there is the opportunity to debate the matter without the pressure of having to make a decision promptly concerning a particular patient. In the future, then, when you call to obtain authorization for such a referral, the medical director knows you and understands how you work and how you came to the decision you did. As a result, the plan has already had the opportunity to explore other options, so a decision can be made promptly—it isn't a surprise.

19. Grievance Procedure

Entering into any business relationship carries with it a certain degree of risk, in the sense that you are now depending upon another party to deliver certain goods or services that you need in order to in turn deliver your product or service. As with any human relationship, there is always the chance that there will be a disagreement, and that disagreement may be serious enough that the two parties may not be able to resolve it themselves. One or both parties may then turn to an outside party—a court or arbitrator—to resolve the dispute.

When looking to resolve a dispute, the objective is to resolve it quickly, fairly, and at minimal cost to the disputants. Turning to the court system by filing a lawsuit against the other party is expensive and time consuming to both parties, and by the nature of a legal action, a lawsuit sharply raises the emotional level of the dispute. Most disputes are simpler and sometimes merely need a formalized system for their resolution.

Many MCOs will have in place a formal system internally to handle disputes once they cannot be resolved informally. There will then be a written policy and procedure outlining how a grievance is filed, who investigates the complaint, and the level of authority to order compliance with the findings. Ask for a copy of the policy, and this policy will be made a part of the contract.

20. Documentation

MCOs may have policy and procedure manuals, newsletters, meetings, and other means of communicating with their providers. Ask what means the MCO uses to communicate with its providers. If there are documents such as procedure manuals, ask to see them at this time. The MCO probably will not allow you to take them or keep them until you sign the contract. It is important, however, that you have an opportunity to review them. In your review, you are looking for anything that will effect your relationship or how you operate. As with other documents, if these are referred to within the contract, they need to be made part of the contract.

21. Required Procedures that Vary from Current Procedures

Managed care contracts impose additional workloads on medical practices—it's just the nature of the beast. In the course of this due diligence review, you've collected a variety of pieces of information as to procedures, forms, and the like that the MCO will be requiring. Now is the time to assess how the MCO's requirements will impact how your practice operates.

One of the key areas to look at is the claims management requirements. Are there any changes that need to be made in your practice management software system in order to accommodate the MCO's requirements? Now is the time to get your vendor involved and make sure that your system can handle the forms, formats, and data sets that are needed to implement and manage the contract.

Most importantly, make sure that your accounting system software can handle capitation plans. A standard accounting system will create an account receivable (A/R) with a service is rendered. When a payment is made, the system will match the payment to the A/R. Capitation payments have not match to A/R, and some systems cannot properly account for it. If your computer system cannot handle capitation, replace the system immediately.

22. Marketing Materials

You will want to see copies of all marketing materials and information being given to members and prospective members. Of particular concern is whether the plan is acting in an ethical manner and, of most importance, whether promises or guarantees are being made which you may not be able to live up to and may be held accountable for.

23. Confirm All Explanations/Agreements in Writing

As with medical records, "If it isn't written, it didn't happen." As you get ready to close your due diligence process, make sure that you have documented explanations and other agreements that you have received from the MCO. Critical issues should be in the form of a letter from the MCO or can be included within the contract.

24. Review Indemnification/Hold Harmless Clause

As noted earlier, this section can be harmless or explosive. The short answer remains—the MCO is responsible for what it does, and you are responsible for what you do.

This is a time to ask about the MCOs liability insurance coverage, which may include a professional liability (malpractice) policy as well. Even with a mutual hold harmless clause, you do want some assurance that you won't get left holding the bag if the MCO defaults on a judgment.

The MCO also may be setting a minimum level of professional liability insurance for your practice to carry. Look for this reference in the contract. If necessary, consult with your insurance carrier to make sure that you meet the requirements of the contract.

25. Legal Review

It is critical that a review be made by an attorney who understands and is familiar with managed care contracts. Your attorney who handles your trust and estate matters is not necessarily this person. Many managed care contracts contain a great deal of language that to an unlearned eye would appear to be not in your best interests. This is a business agreement, and you must understand and be willing to make the trade-offs in order to obtain the agreement.

ANNUAL REVIEW

The next stage in contract management has to do with the annual review. I have come to the belief that as HMOs enter a market area, a good strategy is in fact to sign up with as many as possible and see how the market shakes out. You always have the option later of not renewing an agreement or canceling an agreement by giving the appropriate notice, similar to the rights held by the plan itself. Signing up with as many plans as possible protects you and gives you the option of seeing how the various plans shake out; it also ensures that you are more likely to be retained on a plan's roster as it grows. Getting into a plan that has grown becomes more difficult and you may find yourself locked out.

After you have signed a contract, your evaluation of the MCO does not end. As with any business relationship, you always must be evaluating the relationship as to its value—financial, strategic, and otherwise—to you and your organization. You entered into the contract with certain expectations and assumptions as to performance, patient volume, and revenue. On no less than an annual basis, you should go through a comprehensive review of the MCO and the contract. The key areas to review are outlined below:

1. Volume performance. How many patients are you getting from this plan? Are the demographics in conformance with what you projected? Does utilization conform with your projections? A primary care practice may find a spike in utilization as patients take advantage of the low copayment and catch up on problems that may have been festering. If this is the case, you may find that this will settle down as time goes on.

2. Marketing plans. Has the plan lived up to its projections for growth? Has it achieved its targets for enrollment and employer groups? This also gives you an opportunity to discuss with the plan what its new targets are for the coming year.

3. Public information. You may take a look again at any current filings with the SEC, as well as other filings in your state.

4. The cost of living and consumer price index (CPI). At the time of this writing, the CPI is close to zero, but this of course may change over time. You want to be looking for the current CPI as well as the medical care CPI for your region. This information is available through MGMA and from the regional office of the U.S. Department of Labor.

5. Changes in the local healthcare market. Have practices been merging or folding? Have hospitals been closing, merging, or taken over? Any changes that may have an impact on your practice are what you are looking for, as well as changes that may have an impact on your contract.

6. Changes in the MCO's benefit plan and package. Have there been changes in the MCO's benefit package (i.e., have benefits expanded or contracted)? Of particular note are issues which may impact the services you are providing and whether certain services are now being covered or, conversely, are no longer being covered.

7. Changes in the premium schedules. This is typically public information. If a plan is raising its premiums by 10 percent and proposing to cut your fees, you certainly have grounds to contest its action. You may find that it is surprised that you are aware of the premium increases that they have proposed to the insurance commissioner.

8. Changes in the demographics of the covered population. Is the plan retaining higher or lower risk groups? Many contracts provide that you will accept all patients from any plan or contract that the MCO may enter into. This broad language is fine, on the surface, but lurking in there is the ability for the plan to enter into risk contracts for Medicare and Medicaid patients. Under a fee-for-service system, this usually is not a problem, but under any risk sharing arrangement, there is a problem, unless you are compensated for the difference in utilization. It would not be unusual, for instance, for a capitation rate for a Medicare population to be 2–3 times, or even more, than the capitation rate for a non-Medicare population. In either event, there may then be changes in the utilization of your services.

9. Changes in delivery arrangements. Is the plan adding providers or dropping certain providers with whom you are familiar and utilize on a routine basis? If new arrangements are being made, you may need to obtain new hospital privileges and develop relationships with hospitals and other ancillary providers.

10. Technology and treatment modality changes. These changes can affect your costs as well as the cost of the plan. Lithotripsy, laparoscopic surgery, and the drug TPA are examples of advances that have an impact on your practice and how you get paid. Laparoscopies, for instance, may require more intraoperatory time in surgery, which is a higher cost to you. Therefore, you will want to be paid more by the plan. However, the plan can save significant amounts of money because a laparoscopic procedure may significantly reduce the length of stay. For example, cholecystectomies (gallstone surgery) can cut a hospital length of stay by as much as one-half, even though there is a slight increase in operating room time.

Teleradiography is the newest issue confronting the practice of medicine nationally. The ability of physicians to read radiologic films on a computer enables reading to be done not only down the hall or down the street at the hospital, but across the country if not around the world. How this will be paid for and who will be paid for it are questions that need to be resolved. This is particularly appropriate for tertiary care consultations.

The latest twist on this is telemedicine: the ability to perform certain diagnostic and exam functions via television and telephone lines. There is electronic equipment that enables stethoscope and other physical aspects of an exam to be conducted by a technician with a patient, with the physician watching monitors. Telemedicine raises issues ranging from state licensure for the practice of medicine to how and to whom payment will be made.

Danger Signs

In doing your annual evaluation of a plan, there are several danger signs to look for, including:

1. Decreasing patient panel. If overall the plan is losing members, this obviously is a concern for you, particularly if you are capitated. If the managed care organization is losing market share or key contracts, this is obviously going to have a detrimental effect on your practice and your revenue from the plan. In Georgia, one of the county governments flipped its health insurance coverage with 35,000 covered lives from one carrier to another. If you were a physician in that county and you had a contract with one but not the other plan, you could easily lose upwards of several thousand patients with approximately 30, maybe up to 60, days notice. To avoid becoming overly dependent upon one MCO, you want no more than 20 percent of your revenue coming from one particular HMO.

2. Claims being returned for spurious reasons. In a discussion on claims management, we will discuss ways to follow up on any denial or lack of action, but any inappropriate nonpayment or noncredit for a claim is reason for concern as to the financial health of a plan.

The Due Diligence Checklist presented in this chapter is best used as a basis for developing your own document. Yours, as this one has, will develop and change over time as you gain experience, and as the elements of the contracts change. The data and information collected here is part of building a portrait of the MCO plan, and as the basis for the forthcoming negotiation and subsequent implementation of the contract.

In Chapter 5 there will be further discussion of some of the points of impact on practice operations as a result of MCO contracts.

In the due diligence phase, I recommend that the proposed contract be shared with key staff in the practice and that they be asked for their insights into the impact on operations. These comments will aid the negotiators in identifying and addressing points for discussion with the MCO, and aids the senior management of the practice in ensuring that the practice is prepared to implement the contract in a timely manner without unnecessary problems and obstacles.

3 CHAPTER

Changes in Reimbursement

In the folklore of medicine, physicians were kind men who were dedicated above all else to their patients. They would carry all they needed in the black "doctor's bag," making house calls at all hours of the day or night, delivering babies, caring for sick children and adults alike, and tending to people when they died. Physicians of old were rarely wealthy and were frequently paid "in kind." This could mean chickens, goats, and other kinds of bartered services and products. Television shows such as "Dr. Kildare," "Ben Casey," and, of course, "Marcus Welby, M.D." epitomized this image. My uncle returned from medical school in 1945 and set up his practice in his one room apartment, carved out of the lobby of an apartment building in the Bronx, in New York City. (This was post-World War II, and housing was hard to come by.) When a patient showed up unexpectedly, my aunt and uncle had to fold away the bed and set up the "office."

By the time Medicare and Medicaid were enacted in 1965, health insurance had taken hold throughout the country. More and more citizens were covered, at least in part, by health insurance plans that paid cash to the physicians for services. The post-World War II labor movement frequently sought health insurance coverage for its workers as part of the contract, and large corporations found health insurance to be a relatively inexpensive way to compensate workers.

The Great Society programs of the 1960s and 1970s fueled a great deal of the growth of health care and health care insurance. Programs to serve the elderly, rural communities such as Appalachia, urban programs resulting from the race riots of the 1960s—all had monies earmarked to support health care services. Many of the community health centers, community mental health centers, and rural health clinics originated during these years. In an effort to increase the supply of physicians, and therefore make medical care more accessible, monies flowed to open and expand medical schools, residency training programs, and training programs for nurses and administrators and to build and expand hospitals. One of the oldest federal health initiatives was the Hill–Burton program, passed in 1947. This program provided grants to build and expand hospitals, in return for a guarantee to provide free or reduced fee services to indigent patients.

These programs worked well; so well, in fact, that we are now faced with too many hospitals, too many hospital beds, too many medical schools and medical school slots, too many residency programs, and increasingly, too many physicians (at least in the wrong places).

The funny thing about health care is that it continues to defy the normal "laws" of economics. In spite of the fact that the industry is populated by numerous small providers, all competing with each other, prices tend to remain stable. Historically, pricing information was not available to consumers—consumers never asked, and it was considered unseemly to ask. Patients rarely considered price in the selection of a provider. Health insurance was so popular as an employee benefit that the scope of services covered kept expanding so that employees and their families had to pay few dollars towards their own care. Providers were free to raise their charges because the person making the buying decision (i.e., the person in charge of selecting the provider of the service) was different from the party paying the bill. It was like having a rich uncle who paid all your bills and bailed you out when you got into trouble.

Interestingly, the first Blue Cross plans were formed in the 1930s as a means for hospitals to insure that they would be paid.

Hospitalization was a much more serious event than it is today, and the financial needs were catastrophic in nature—hence the need and practicality of insurance.

The Blue Cross story began in 1929 when Justin Ford Kimball, an official at Baylor University in Dallas, Texas, introduced a plan to guarantee school teachers 21 days of hospital care for the grand sum of $6 a year. The idea quickly spread through Texas and into Iowa and Illinois. By 1935, there were 15 plans in 11 states, and most began to adopt the "blue cross" symbol that had been devised by an executive of the Minnesota plan in 1933. In 1936, the American Hospital Association formed the Committee on Hospital Services to coordinate these plans, which required state legislation in order to support the not-for-profit status of the plans. By 1960, Blue Cross plans insured almost one-third of the U.S. population, and the name was becoming synonymous with health insurance.

The 1990s have brought dramatic changes to the Blue Cross plans. Changes in the health care world have driven some plans to merge and others to declare bankruptcy. Anthem, the Blue Cross licensee in Indiana and parts of Kentucky and Illinois, has merged with New Jersey Blue Cross (which in turn had merged with the Delaware plan only a week earlier). The Mountain State (West Virginia) Blue Cross crashed, and Empire Blue Cross (downstate New York) was ridden by scandal and huge losses. The number of plans has shrunk from 78 to 67 in the last decade alone.

The Blue Shield plans grew out of the lumber and mining camps of the Pacific Northwest at the turn of the century. In the tradition of employer paternalism, arrangements were made with local physicians to pay a monthly fee for their services. In 1917, physicians around Tacoma, Washington, and Pierce County created a "medical services bureau" to provide these services. These bureaus became the basis of the Blue Shield Plans, some of which still operate today. In 1982, the Blue Cross Association and the National Association of Blue Shield Plans merged to become the Blue Cross and Blue Shield Association. Headquartered in Chicago, the association controls the license of the name and symbols, and it has licensees in all 50 states, the District of Columbia, Puerto Rico, Australia, Canada, Jamaica, and the United Kingdom. The plans serve some 86 million beneficiaries of the private and Medicare services.

In the 1990s, health insurance is driven not by the needs of the providers, but by the needs of the people footing the bill—employers and government (the "buyers"). Slowly over time the buyers have begun to *act* as buyers, negotiating prices, using market power to obtain discounts, standardizing purchases and limiting supplier options, and demanding and evaluating the quality of services rendered. Even today, physicians and other providers are having trouble dealing with the notion that they have to be accountable for what they do.

The world of the 1990s is very different. Reimbursement used to be a simple affair: see the patient, bill the insurance company your charge, and require the patient to pay some portion. Today, most physician practice revenue is governed by a managed care or direct contracting arrangement. The payer, more importantly, may turn out not to be an insurance company, but actually another physician group practice, a hospital, a physician–hospital organization (PHO), or some other noninsurance company creature. Increasingly, employers and health plans are simply turning over a piece of the premium dollar to one provider entity, and it is that provider entity that is going out, perhaps building a provider network (which may be its own organization), and even sharing a piece of the premium with the new organization. It's often compared to the food chain from your high school biology class; the smaller fish hang around the bigger fish looking for the scraps that the bigger fish don't bother to eat.

Today, employers fight with payers, payers fight with providers, providers fight with payers and each other; reimbursement for health care services has been reduced to a scramble over the health insurance premium dollar. Chapter 4, "Capitation," will discuss the consolidation of contracting and the outsourcing of provider networks, financing, and service provisions by the health plans to large, integrated (real or virtual) provider organizations.

Medical practices of today do not truly operate according to the retail model of a service rendered and cash collected. Unlike most businesses, cash is not collected at the time the service is rendered. Rather, practices must bill their services to a health plan, thus carrying large accounts receivable on their books until the plan reimburses some portion of the charge. Practices grant discounts by "accepting assignment," that is, accepting the payment from the patient's health plan as payment in full and writing off the difference, or then billing a secondary carrier or the patient for the balance due.

Contracting with managed care plans, however, is different. Fundamental to health maintenance organizations (HMOs) and preferred provider organizations (PPOs) is the notion that there will be no balance billing. Billing an indemnity carrier is like rolling the dice—one never truly knows what will be paid, regardless of any history with the carrier for the same service. MCO contracts, however, come with a specified fee schedule for the services to be rendered.

As we've moved toward a buyer-driven market, a number of new and innovative reimbursement schemes have been developed. The 1960s saw the enactment of Medicare and the Medicare acts and the growth of usual and customary reimbursement (UCR). UCR fees were set by insurance companies based upon a profile which they would develop based upon the actual physician billings. Insurance companies also had the ability to capture fee information from similar specialties in geographic areas defined by the companies. There were no clear-cut models or any rules of how these UCR fees were set, and some would even speculate that the fees were somewhat random and arbitrary in how they were established. Needless to say, the insurance industry would not share this information with providers.

But no matter. Fee for service by and large is rapidly declining, although it is far from dead. A more common model these days is the negotiated fee, whereby the insurance carrier, managed care plan, or broker will negotiate a reduced fee in return for the promise of directing a new flow of patients to the physician. In the case of Medicare there is no negotiation, but there is a reduced fee, based upon the resource based relative value units (RBRVU).

Today, there are about eight ways health providers are being paid. The traditional means is fee for service; much the way other professions are paid for their services, a set fee is determined for what the professional does for the client or patient. Health care, however, has moved away from fee for service as the sole method. There continues to be experimentation with a variety of reimbursement schemes that seek to hold the professional (the physician) accountable and responsible for the quantity, quality, and cost of all health care services, not just physician services, that are rendered for a patient. The various reimbursement schemes all use money as both a carrot and a stick to induce physicians to change their patterns of using services. Use outpatient and primary care services, get an extra check. Use the hospital, have some money taken away. The conundrum that faces employers and payers is determining which incentives, or combination of incentives, will insure that a patient gets only the care that he needs, but also all of the care that he needs. That is another debate and another book, and it doesn't help you with the here and now.

The eight methods for provider reimbursement being used at this writing include:[1]

1. Outcome based pricing
2. Capitation
3. Risk pool/withhold
4. Case rate
5. Episode rate
6. Per diem
7. Discounted fee for service
8. Fee for service

This list moves from the highest degree of risk to the provider to the lowest degree of risk (defining risk as the expense and work effort the provider will have to expend without a linkage to revenue). Each type of payment scheme has a different means of incentives for providers.

- **Outcome-based pricing.** This type of payment scheme involves a fee paid to achieve a specific outcome. An example of outcome-based pricing would be a transplant, where an organ rejection within a certain time frame would necessitate the facility and the transplant team to do a second procedure, all for a single price.

[1]The discussion in this section is based on Alison Cherney, *The Capitation & Risk Sharing Guidebook* (Burr Ridge, IL: Irwin Professional Publishing, 1996), p. 5.

- **Capitation.** Capitation involves a predetermined payment for each member of a health plan assigned to a provider for a defined set of services. Payment is usually made on a monthly basis.
- **Risk pool/withhold.** This method can be used in conjunction with other forms, usually discounted fee-for-service arrangements. A certain amount of the fee is set aside in a pool, and it is only distributed to providers if certain performance standards (utilization of services or certain services) are met.
- **Episode rate.** These rates are developed when it is difficult to predict the length of a case but the service required and the length of the episode can be quantified.
- **Case rate.** This method provides an all-inclusive rate for a case; most commonly, it is used for a procedure to cover all professional, facility, and ancillary charges. An example would be a case rate for a coronary arterial bypass graft (CABG).
- **Per diem.** This is a fixed daily rate for the services provided. It is commonly used for hospital reimbursement.
- **Discounted fee for service.** This may be the most common form of reimbursement. The payer negotiates a discount from the provider's standard full fee schedule.
- **Fee for service.** This is the traditional means of payment, in which a fee is paid for each specific service.

For physicians' practices, three of the eight payment schemes are most commonly used: discounted fee for service; withhold and risk pool; and capitation.

Fee for service remains the most common model for payment by far. More than 60 percent of physician services are paid on a fee for service (albeit discounted fee for service) basis. What began as straightforward fees, which patients paid in cash or in trade, has slowly been eroding in the post-World War II years. Since the war, health insurance plans have surged, covering an increasingly greater portion of the population. For many larger employers, providing for generous health insurance was a relatively inexpensive means of increasing employee compensation when compared to wage increases. Labor unions often seized on health insurance as a bargaining tool as well, seeking ever-increasing benefits and the extension of coverage to retirees.

The setting of professional fees is often based on less than sound methodologies. Many practices set their fees when the physician hangs up his shingle, and then they methodically increase them across the board by some percentage, often tied to the consumer price index, over the years. The result is a fee schedule that may not be reflective of either market rates or the changing cost of providing different services. When you get a fee schedule from a managed care plan, you may be very shocked to see some of the rates being offered—"Look at all the money I'm losing"—but in fact you may still be very profitable.

RISK AND REIMBURSEMENT

As we've been discussing, central to the notion of managed care is the insurance concept of risk. Risk is the probability of a given event occurring. Risk for trading a stock on the stock exchange means one thing, while risk for the purposes of insurance means another, and risk for providers means yet something else. Before moving into the discussion of withholds and risk pools and capitation, it is important to understand the fundamentals of risk in the context of physician practice management.

Among the first examples of insurance is Lloyd's of London, the venerable "insurer of last resort." Lloyd's was founded in a coffee house on the London docks, where shipowners could insure their ships against sinking or attack. The idea behind insurance is that of shared risk. Every shipowner was at risk that his ship would sink and he would suffer a "loss." But although all owners were at risk of loss, in reality, not all would suffer loss—only some would. By forming an insurance pool, gathering together funds from a large number of owners, all would share the cost of the few ships that sank. The payment, the premium, was less than the cost of a lost ship and cargo and, more importantly, was a predictable expense.

On a daily basis, most people are familiar with insurance, most commonly with home owner and auto insurance policies. In daily life there is the risk that there will be a monetary loss to a person through the loss of property from fire, flood, or storm, the loss of business equipment, the loss of earning power due to injury or illness, or the need to satisfy very expensive obligations due to personal actions or some untoward event. The idea behind insurance is that all parties have varying degrees of risk that they will incur a claim in the course of a year. This group of people, often referred to as "covered lives," will band together and pay money into a fund (the insurance company), which acts as a trust. This insurance organization, or trust, will then pay people who have a claim in the course of a year. Those who do not have a claim will not get their money back. The idea is that by paying for insurance through the premium, a person (or company) has essentially fixed the risk of his loss from such an event. Insurance protects a person from being severely damaged or wiped out financially from such a loss.

The same concept applies to an automobile insurance policy. Although many states require certain minimum amounts of insurance, individuals can choose to buy more expensive coverage: that is, coverage which will pay a higher amount of losses. One does not insure for an unlimited amount of money. In other words, there are limits to how much your auto policy will pay in the event of a loss. More importantly, there is a minimum as well. The deductible, which we are familiar with, is essentially a provision whereby the insured has taken on the risk for a portion of the loss. If your deductible is $250, your premium is much higher than the person who has a deductible of $1,000. The reason for this is that the likelihood, that is, the risk, of a claim with a loss of greater than $250 is much higher than an accident wherein the loss is greater than $1,000. For the first $250 the individual is responsible, and the insurance company will pay from $251 up to the maximum of the policy. Under the second scenario with a higher deductible, the insurance company does not pay a penny until the loss amounts to over $1,000. The likelihood of the carrier having to pay under a $1,000 deductible is much less; therefore, the risk is much less and the premium charged the insured is much less as well.

Insurance companies have their own insurance companies that insure against such losses. Although one or a group of carriers may be responsible for all the claims, these companies factor in the likelihood of such an event really happening. Although they have accepted the risk, the risk is small enough that they then turn to what are known as reinsurance companies to cover heavy losses or, more importantly, heavier-than-expected losses for the whole company in a given year. Incidents such as an earthquake or a major hurricane in the course of one year are all events that could have a major impact on the viability of the insurance company.

One of the principals underlying paradigms of the insurance industry is the need to convey that the insurance company is stable and will be in business should someone have a claim. In health insurance the insurance carrier must predict as much as 18 or more months in advance how much money it will be paying out to individuals and providers for claims made. The limits of a policy under health plans are typically very high, usually subject to a lifetime maximum of $1 to $2 million dollars. The actuaries, whose job it is to predict utilization, often work with fuzzy and somewhat inaccurate data and are essentially making a projection or forecast of events that will happen far in the future.

Two major reimbursement methods—withholds / risk pools and capitation—both rely on the transfer of some of the risk of paying for medical losses as a means of incentive to the physician. Risk pools link the incentive, a cash payment, to performance; that is, utilization that meets or exceeds the target budget. Capitation transfers the cost of care, rather than the price, to the provider, who then makes the decisions as to when to spend resources in services or when to withhold it. In both scenarios, if the physician is able to limit utilization to the projected targets, he has a higher profit to keep for himself.

WITHHOLDS AND RISK POOLS

Withholds and risk pools are fee-for-service based, but with twists. In simple terms, the payer is paying the provider on a negotiated fee-for-service schedule but withholds a certain percentage (often 20 percent) from each payment during the course of a year. While risk withholds may have their origin in discounted fee-for-service settings, they also can appear in capitation and other arrangements. Let's walk through an example, using a discounted fee-for-service arrangement, to show the principles of this method.

Steps to Withhold: An Example

Suppose that the physician group estimates services for Chuck's HMO for the coming year as follows:

Number of units of service:	2,500
Average fee per unit:	$100
Estimated revenue	$250,000

However, there will be a "20 percent withhold," meaning that 20 percent of the fee schedule fees will be held back by the HMO. These monies will be placed into a fund known as a "risk pool."

At the end of the year, the actual numbers are as follows:

Number of units of service:	2,750
Average collected fee per unit:	$80
Gross revenue:	$275,000
Less: 20 percent withheld:	($55,000)
Net revenue / cash collection:	$220,000

The practice has exceeded the budget target by 10 percent, or $27,500. These monies are then subtracted from the monies in the risk pool as follows:

$55,000 in risk pool	
Less: $25,000 overrun	
Net remaining in risk pool:	$30,000

Since there are still monies remaining in the risk pool, the remaining monies are distributed to the physician practice. A check is cut and sent to the practice for $27,500. The total revenue is as follows:

Net cash collections during year:	$220,000
Plus: Risk pool distribution:	$30,000
Total cash collections:	$250,000

Average collection per unit of service: $250,000 divided by 2,750 units of service = $90.91 / unit of service

Now, many readers will look at the $90.91 average collection per unit and compare that to the $100 per unit fee, a fee that is already discounted, and recoil in horror. But all may not be as it appears.

The practice had a contract for an average fee of $100 per unit of service, less a risk pool withhold that could amount to as much as 20 percent of that. Is this a good contract? A bad contract? An OK contract? Or a run-of-the mill contract? To answer this question, one needs to compare the revenue under the risk pool withhold to the actual collections under similar scenarios.

In comparing fees, there is one calculation that is often forgotten: adjusting the fee by the collection rate to account for bad debt, contractual allowances, and other uncollectables. These often can total 20 to 30 percent of the full fee. But a word of caution here: a collection rate is only meaningful in relation to itself within one practice over a period of time. Further, that relationship assumes a steady state. I once put in an imaging service in an internal medicine practice, and the collection rate fell by over 10 percent. This had nothing to do with the effectiveness of the billing and collection staff. It had everything to do with a big ticket service that was steeply discounted by Medicare and certain other payers. Since this was anticipated in planning the service, it was not a surprise nor a problem.

The following worksheet presents how to perform a comparison. First, set up a spreadsheet as displayed below (Table 3–1) and enter the following data:

Step 1: Enter all (CPT) codes used by the practice.

Step 2: Enter your "private" fee schedule by code.

Step 3: Enter your utilization by code for the current year.

Step 4: Compute your gross revenue (utilization multiplied by fee).

Step 5: Adjust by collection rate to determine net cash collections.

Step 6: Determine total units of service from the current year.

Step 7: Divide net cash collections (from Step 5) by total units of service (from Step 6) to determine average net cash collections per unit of service.

The next step is to do the same calculation under the discounted fee-for-service. The final set of calculations under a risk pool system is as follows:

Step 8: Enter net cash collections paid to practice during the year $__________

TABLE 3–1

CPT Code	Full Fee	Utilization	Gross Revenue
Step 1. Enter all CPT codes for your practice	**Step 2.** Enter your fee schedule	**Step 3.** Enter utilization data	**Step 4.** Multiply fee times utilization
Example: 99232	*$55.00*	*350*	*$19,250.00*
			Step 5: Multiply (90%) by collection rate to determine net cash collections
		Step 6: Determine total units of service	**Step 7:** Divide total net cash collections by total units of service
		Example: 350	*$49.50*

The next step is to do the same calculation under the discounted fee for service:

CPT Code	Discounted Fee	Utilization	Gross Revenue
Step 8: Enter all CPT codes for your practice	**Step 9:** Enter your discounted fee schedule	**Step 10:** Enter utilization data	**Step 11:** Fee times utilization
Example: 99232	*$50.00*	*350*	*$17,500.00*
	Less: 20% withhold		**Step 12:** Adjust by 20% withhold
Example:	*$40.00*	*350*	*$14,400.00*

Step 13: Add the risk pool distribution settlement $________

Step 14: Add the numbers from Step 12 and Step 13 to determine total cash collections for the year: $________

Step 15: Divide the total cash collections (from Step 14) by the total units of service for the year (from Step 6) to determine the average collections per unit of service: $________

Step 16: Compare the average net collections per unit of service (from Step 15) with the average net cash collections per unit of service (from Step 7). Difference $________ or ________%

Under the risk pool payment system, the key factor to consider is the *average cash collections per unit of service.* This is your real fee. As the level of discounting, fixed fee, prepayments, and other nonfee service arrangements increase, your real fee decreases. The analogy is a department store that is always running sales; the "full" price becomes a fiction, because fewer people actually pay it. Wait a minute, and the item will be on sale again.

The determinant of success is the profit per unit. Under a risk withhold system, you will receive the negotiated fee less the withhold. For every unit of service you deliver, you will be paid that net fee, regardless of the quantity of services. It is possible to achieve higher dollar profits by continuing to generate services. However, you still have the variable cost of performing the service, and your return on investment is still declining. The incentive here is to increase your profit per unit of service.

SELF INSURANCE

As with any insurance, the more risk that the insured can assume, the lower the premium. For large employers, they can save significant amounts of money by self-insuring for their employees' health benefits. When self-insured, the company pays all claims from its own pocket. It may purchase a "stop loss" policy, which may be as simple as a policy with a very high deductible. Even organizations with as few as 50 employees can save considerably on their health insurance premiums by self-insuring for high deductible amounts. (There is a big caveat here: you also must purchase a "stop loss" policy in the event of catastrophic illness. While an option, do proceed cautiously!)

For large employers, they will assume all of the risk for health benefit payments. In these situations, a large organization such as IBM or Xerox may hire what is known as a third party administrator (TPA). Very often, the TPA organization is an insurance carrier such as Prudential or an HMO such as HealthSource, and it will handle the claims management for the employer. In most states, TPA companies are licensed by the state insurance department. Patients and even providers, many times, are confused and do not understand that they may be dealing with a TPA rather than a regular indemnity plan, for example. This TPA may even have the power to negotiate contracts, develop networks, and generally function much like a managed care plan functions absent the direct insurance carrier activities.

Over the past few years, employers have been moving away from the standard indemnity type arrangements and inducing their employees to move into managed care plans. Many have moved in several steps, beginning by setting up financial incentives for employees who choose the managed care plans. For example, the employee portion of the premium is often much lower (if there is an employee portion at all) when the MCO is selected as opposed to choosing the indemnity plan. Over time, however, some companies have begun to eliminate the indemnity plans and mandate managed care coverage. In 1995, for example, AT&T moved all 40,000 managers in its New Jersey headquarters, plus another 60,000 dependents, into a U.S. Healthcare HMO plan. With a health care bill of $1 billion annually (equal to 20 percent of its annual profits) AT&T had a powerful incentive to act decisively.

Larger employers now are beginning to move beyond managed care and are bypassing the health plans entirely. Rather than contracting with MCOs to administer the provider network, these employers are going directly to the providers to set up contracts. Now, direct contracting is nothing new; large employers have had contracts whereby the provider was paid directly on a fee-for-service basis for services rendered to the employer's covered lives. What we are now seeing in areas such as Cleveland, Minneapolis, and Southern California is that employers are contracting directly with providers on a risk sharing basis. Rather than paying the carrier to administer the "premium" dollars, the buyers are going to the providers and saying, "Here's the pool of premium dollars. Take care of our employees and dependents." The employers are leaving it to the providers to sort out how to divvy up the dollars.

Minneapolis has a very interesting experiment underway as this is written. A consortium of large employers, organized into the Buyers' Health Care Action Group (BHCAG), has issued requests for proposal (RFPs) to provide for hospital and physician services for their employees. BHCAG is seeking responses from what it calls "care systems." Care systems consist of: a hospital (or hospitals), primary care physicians, and specialty physicians. Primary care physicians can only affiliate with one care system, while specialists can affiliate with more than one care system. BHCAG, in turn, will pay the care systems on a fee-for-service basis and then leave it up to the care systems to divvy up the monies. The next step in the plan, it is speculated, is that the BHCAG will hand over a given amount of money—a health care budget (remember those?)—and tell the care system, "Take care of our employees and dependents." Employees will get a voucher from their employer which will have a value, perhaps for the lowest cost plan or care system. If the employee chooses a higher cost care system, the employer may only pay a portion or none of the incremental cost.

In several places in the country, most famously perhaps the MedPartners/Mullikan Group in Southern California, providers are taking entering into risk contracts directly with employers. By taking on risk contracts directly from the buyers, however, the providers are then acting like an insurance company, taking in a fixed amount of monies (a premium) in return for ensuring that all needed services will be provided. In the Mullikan situation, the State of California has ruled that it must obtain a license as an insurance company/HMO in order to enter into these types of agreements.

Nationally, there has been a mixture of responses by state regulatory agencies. The National Association of Insurance Commissioners (NAIC) has issued a position paper stating that these types of arrangements are insurance functions and, as such, fall under the police powers of the state and need to be regulated as insurance companies. NAIC has developed the "Consolidated Licenser of Entities Accepting Risk Model Act" (CLEAR) and is seeking passage by the states.

One of the requirements of state insurance laws and CLEAR is that organizations that assume risk in a direct contracting situation must meet a number of requirements, particularly the maintenance of financial reserves. There were proposals in Congress in 1996, part of the "deal" between the Republican majority and the American Medical Association, that would have allowed provider sponsored organizations to deliver services under Medicare managed care arrangements without the state insurance licensure requirements, most importantly, the requirements for financial reserves. Financial reserves are a very important consideration, as anyone who has had to recover a claim filed with a bankrupt insurance company can testify. (I once had to do it—my hospital recovered just 10 percent of the policy coverage.)

Large organizations will be able to go the Mullikan route, obtain their state insurance company licenses, and enter directly into risk bearing contracts with employers. The Minneapolis model offers some fascinating possibilities for providers and physician groups. This model does not require the formation of large integrated organizations, but instead it allows hospitals and physicians to work together, perhaps through a joint venture organization such as a PHO. Joint ventures (JV) are a faster way to initiate structural changes within an industry, since JVs don't require a formal, legal merger in order for the partners to work together. JVs such as PHOs also allow the various players to remain independent and delay having to deal with the numerous control and other issues of hospitals acquiring medical practices.

With all the changes in reimbursement schemes, new types of organizations, mergers, consolidations, and general turmoil, when the smoke clears, there are really only a few key issues. One is the demand on the part of buyers and payers that we as providers demonstrate that what we do for patients—all the tests, procedures, prescriptions, and the like—makes a difference and that what we are doing we are doing well. Secondly, payers want prices to come down. It sometimes looks like the payers are tossing a bone (premium dollars) at the providers and watching while we scramble to get as much of the electronic transfers as we can for ourselves.

Risk withholds, full risk capitation (see the next chapter), direct contracting to care systems—all of these are mechanisms whereby insurance companies or buyers are simply handing over portions of the premium dollars to providers and telling them, "Here it is—you divvy it up and leave us out of it." As you will see further in this book, the fight we wage is over who will get the premium dollars—hospitals, care systems, integrated delivery systems, physician practice management companies, large, multispecialty group practices, or even insurance companies.

4 CHAPTER

Capitation

Capitation has been around for over 50 years, but it is only in the last few years that we have seen it become a major method of payment for medical practices. It is the most misunderstood of the payment schemes and poses a high level of risk to physician groups. It is not, however, the death knell of medical practices, and many practices find that they do well under capitation contracts.

It still amazes me the degree of misinformation and disinformation that exists surrounding capitation. Capitation in and of itself is neither good nor bad. Some practices do very well with capitation; some have trouble. Capitation does not mean you the physician are working for or are an employee of a health plan, nor does it mean you are being paid not to deliver care.

As with everything else in health care, as soon as a concept takes hold, it mutates into a variety of new forms. Some are good. Some are scourges and should be eradicated from the earth. In this chapter, I will first discuss "simple" capitation: an HMO pays one provider a capitation fee for the services for which the provider, and only the provider, is responsible. I will also discuss "full risk medical capitation," where a group is responsible for providing or paying for all professional physician services needed for their patients, regardless of who provides the service or where the service is provided.

The origins of capitation go back to the Great Depression era. Sidney Garfield, a young surgeon, was running a 12-bed Contractors General Hospital in the Mojave Desert to serve the thousands of workers building the Los Angeles Aqueduct.[1] Having trouble collecting from insurance companies and uninsured workers, Garfield ran into financial problems. An engineer turned insurance agent named Harold Hatch suggested that insurance companies pay a fixed sum of money per day per covered worker up front. The initial rate was five cents per day per worker, and for an additional five cents per day, a worker also could be covered for nonjob related medical problems. Thus was born "prepayment." The plan was a success, and Garfield and his hospital prospered.

After the aqueduct project wound down, Garfield was approached by industrialist Henry Kaiser to do the same thing for the workers and their dependents building the Grand Coulee Dam. Garfield upgraded his hospital and recruited several physicians to join him in his venture. In 1941, as the dam project was completed, World War II was gearing up, and Kaiser called upon Garfield to replicate his program for the workers at the Kaiser shipyards in Richmond, California. It was only after the war ended that the plan, named the Permanente Health Plan, was opened to the public and began the steady growth that eventually made what is now known as the Kaiser Permanente Health Plan the largest health maintenance organization (HMO) in the country. (For more information about Kaiser, see its web site at www.kaiplan.com.)

Similar to the Blue Cross plans, the Kaiser plan was founded as a means of providing a steady and reliable cash flow to hospitals—Contractors General in the case of Kaiser, and Baylor Hospital in Houston, Texas, in the case of Blue Cross. The original notion was simple and direct: prepayment for all medical services. The belief system and incentive was to promote a healthful lifestyle and preventative medicine, thereby reducing the need for medical care. This notion has been all too forgotten or bastardized by too many of the newer plans and providers scrambling to save

---

[1]Kaiser Permanente, *50 Years of Quality,* (Oakland, CA: Kaiser Foundation Health Plan. Web Site, 1996).

their organizations and their jobs. As you will see, perhaps returning to the roots of what we call managed care is the key to success in the world of today.

But first, let's walk through how capitation works, the incentives, and the strategies and motivations of the payers and providers. Finally, let's follow the money.

I hear too often the cry, "My incentive under capitation is not to see patients." The response to that? "Turn in your license." What capitation means is that you, the physician, are being paid regardless of whether or not you deliver care. Let me suggest the analogy of life insurance. Life insurance companies heavily market the case stories of how, when the family breadwinner died, there was the life insurance company with the check for the proceeds of the policy. The survivors then had money to bury their loved one and pay their living expenses. If life insurance policies never paid off, then why in the world would anyone buy them? If physicians accept capitation monies but don't see patients, why should employers and employees buy health insurance for physician care?

Capitation can be compared to a retainer, almost like a coverage for standby costs. From a business perspective the concept is simple: the health plan is paying you a set amount of money to effectively reserve a given block of your time to care for its members—your patients. Sometimes you will be able to do this in the course of the amount of time you have set aside, and other times you will have to spend more than that time. In either event, you are being paid to "stand by."

Capitation is defined as a payment for a defined scope of services for a defined population set (covered lives) for a defined period of time. Capitation payments are a fixed amount of money, a dollar amount, paid to the provider each month for each person for which the provider is responsible for providing services. This is known as per member per month, or PMPM. When you negotiate a capitation rate, what you are negotiating is the PMPM. So for each member from the health plan who has selected you as his provider, you will be paid that given PMPM. If you are a specialist it is more likely that you will be paid an amount based upon the whole membership in the plan or the membership in a given geographic region.

That's how capitation works in practice. But why is capitation so attractive to managed care organizations (MCOs)? What capitation does is shift risk—risk of paying claims and the risk of adjudicating claims—from the insurance companies to the providers. HMOs are the versions of MCOs that can offer risk contracts, and HMOs are first and foremost insurance companies. As insurance companies, HMOs have several roles:

- Develop insurance products and market these products to employers and individuals.
- Collect premiums.
- Administer preauthorization and utilization management programs.
- Receive, process, and pay claims.

In his book, *Capitation: New Opportunities in Healthcare Delivery*, capitation expert David Samuels suggests that HMOs simply are not equipped to handle the complexity of managing health care claims and find it cheaper and easier to "outsource" the utilization management and claims adjudication functions to providers.[2] Samuels suggests that HMOs don't adjudicate claims; they simply process and pay what is received based upon a set of sometimes Byzantine and fuzzy rules and procedures. Unlike traditional forms of insurance, such as general liability and property and casualty, HMOs do not undertake any substantial effort to manage and reduce the risk of claims. Property and casualty insurance underwriting has a heavy emphasis on prevention, exemplified in the insurance industry's push for building and fire codes. The first fire departments in this country were set up by insurance companies which placed "fire marks" (small metal emblems noting the insurance company) on the sides of buildings that the company insured. Even today, some property owners in New York City will find the New York Fire Patrol responding to some building fires. The Fire Patrol, run by a group of insurance companies, is responsible for protecting interior property from fire and water damage and salvaging property after the fire is under control.

---

[2]For an excellent, detailed discussion of capitation and where it is going, see David Samuels, *Capitation: New Opportunities in Healthcare Delivery* (Burr Ridge, IL: Irwin Professional Publishing, 1996).

But where, Samuels asks, are the insurance companies when it comes to preventing and limiting claims in the health insurance setting? Nowhere. Instead, they have simply outsourced those responsibilities, transferring them to the providers, who are also ill-equipped to address them, or simply don't want to or don't know how to. As I have also been a proponent of this approach to managing capitation, see Chapter 9 for a discussion of health education and prevention.

So, faced with two forces, an inability to carry out traditional insurance functions in health care, and a rapid increase in the utilization and cost of services, HMOs respond by transferring risk and stopping their own losses by fixing in advance the amount they pay to providers. In effect, they take a portion of the insurance premium they are receiving from employers and pay that portion, and only that portion, to providers. What has happened is that the payer is effectively saying to the provider, "Look, since you control the utilization and therefore what I/we will be paying, you the provider need to take responsibility for what this costs." In insurance jargon, the claims paid are referred to as "medical losses." The percentage of total premiums that are paid out is known as the "medical loss ratio." Some critics of managed care have used this as a means of attacking the plans, noting that they regard people's medical care needs as a loss. In fact, these are simply common insurance terms, that is, someone has experienced a loss that entails a monetary loss (due to illness in this case as opposed to a loss due to damage to a house or an automobile accident).

Now that providers are taking on risk, it is important to understand what that risk is composed of. The transfer of risk means the provider will be responsible for some of these losses.[3] There are three elements that provide a risk: (1) underpricing risk; (2) fluctuation risk; and (3) business risk.

For underpricing risk, the risk is that a provider will not charge enough or have a high enough PMPM to cover its costs and make a sufficient profit. A smaller profit margin leaves less room for error. Under capitation and all managed care plans, what happens is that revenue to a provider typically but not always does go down, leaving smaller profit margins and less room for

---

[3]Bruce S. Pyenson, Editor, *Calculated Risk: A Provider's Guide to Assessing and Controlling the Financial Risk of Managed Care* (Chicago, IL: American Hospital Publishing, Inc., 1995).

error in the management of the organization. Operating costs often also rise in proportion to the rise in managed care volume, putting further pressure on profits.

Underpricing is driven by three types of "service" risk to providers:

1. *Frequency.* The overall utilization of services by the MCO's members exceeds the projections.
2. *Intensity.* The volume and mix of services exceeds the projections.
3. *Cost.* The average cost of providing services exceeds the projections.

Fluctuation risk is a random or unlucky event. I live in coastal South Carolina where, at this writing, State Farm and Nationwide will not write homeowner's policies. The reason is simple. The risk of a hurricane (and in some parts, the risk of earthquake) is high enough that there is a higher risk that there will be a catastrophe in this area than, say, the Midwest, at least from a hurricane. In 1992, Hurricane Andrew in Florida, combined with a California earthquake, left many insurance carriers scrambling for monies to pay the tremendous losses incurred that year. The year before and the year after, losses were in the "usual range" or perhaps even lower than usual, and the insurers may have been making money. However, all it takes is that bad year. In the case of Nationwide, reportedly it had written so many policies in coastal South Carolina that it felt it could not take on any more because if there were another hurricane, the claims would far exceed the firm's ability to make payment. It has thus limited its risk by stopping and fixing a dollar amount of property which it will cover.

The third type of risk is business risk. Business risk has to do with the day-to-day risk we have in doing business. For physician groups, business risk has three principal components: (1) The stability of the health plan to ensure that it will continue to make the claims payments and capitation payments; (2) the ability of the provider to collect the copayment and coinsurance amounts required; and (3) the general risk in running a business in today's world.

Any one or a combination of the above risks are what face the physician practice in a capitation situation. Upon entering into the initial contract with the MCO, the physician practice assumes a certain degree of business risk. A price is set to pay for the services that the practice will provide to a group of MCO members. A projection is made as to the amount of services that the practice will provide in the course of the year. If the volume of services far exceeds the projection, the practice has underpriced its services. If the variation is a "fluctuation" (a flu epidemic, for example), this is dealt with one way. On the other hand, if the original utilization assumptions are markedly off actual experience, the practice's services have been underpriced.

One question that I hear frequently concerning capitation is: What's a good rate? And the answer, the reason why you're reading this book, is . . . it depends. It depends on several factors, the most important one being: What services are covered under this capitation contract and rate? Am I only responsible for the service my group provides? Am I responsible for all professional services my group provides but no services related to diagnostic procedures? Am I responsible for all professional services, either provided by my group, in the emergency department, or by specialists outside of my group (for which I have approved the referral)? Am I responsible for any facility or ancillary service charges? In order to assess the capitation rate, you must first clarify the "degree of capitation" being proposed; that is, how extensive are the scope of services to be covered by the rate?

Some terminology will be helpful at this point:

- *Partial risk medical capitation rate.* Covers only those services covered by defined professionals, usually the members of an independent practice association (IPA) or group practice. Which providers and which services are covered under the capitation rate must be clearly spelled out in the contract.
- *Full risk medical capitation rate.* Paid to the group to cover all medical professional services, whether primary care or specialty care, wherever the service is delivered—office, hospital, or outpatient center. If your group receives the full risk capitation payment, you often are responsible for receiving the claims from the other providers and paying those claims.

FIGURE 4–1

Premium Allocation under Full Risk Capitation

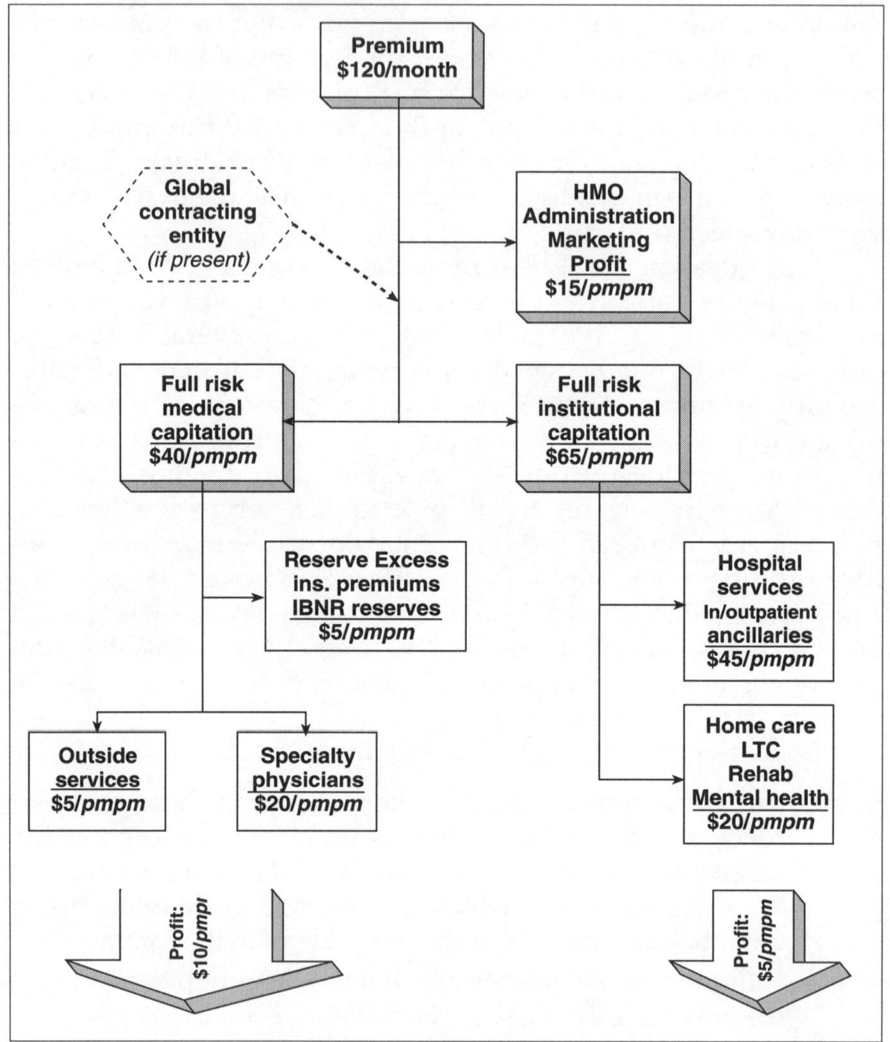

- *Full risk institutional capitation rate.* Paid to a hospital or other organization to cover all facility fees for inpatient and outpatient hospital, rehab services, mental health, and other alternative site providers.

- *Global or full risk capitation rate.* Paid to an organization to cover all professional medical as well as all facility fees. The fees due to the providers are paid by the contracting entity. Responsibility for overall utilization management, quality assurance, and marketing may reside with the contracting entity or with the health plan.

At this writing, the more common scenario is partial medical risk capitation, where the HMO pays a medical group a capitation rate for the services that the group provides. Referrals to specialists are subject to approval by the HMO, and it is the HMO that has the risk and financial responsibility for paying the specialists.

Usually, faced with a capitation contract, the physician will ask, "How do I know if I'm making money or not?" There are several methods to set your capitation price and to evaluate proposals from MCO plans. Before we deal with that question, let's round out the understanding of capitation with some background discussion on risk.

To say that this is an inexact science is an understatement. Health care also has been subject to very fast growth in the utilization and costs of services which makes projections more difficult to make. As a result, premium increases have been in double digits over the past years as insurers have had to both play catch up as well as build reserves to pay out future claims.

The MCO has to project utilization of services in order to establish the premium that it will be charging employers for health insurance coverage. Capitation plans are one way to transfer some of the risk of paying for services onto the provider. There are usually limits to this risk, however, so the MCO still needs to insure that utilization is controlled. The key to running any managed care plan is the ability to control utilization. It's that simple. As a friend of mine who was the medical director of an HMO said, "Utilization begins in the physician's office." Once the physician has picked up the phone to make a referral, money has been spent.

This having been said, some of the key success factors under capitation include the ability to do the right thing, do it right (quality), and manage it well. It is a matter of value rather than the lowest cost. Remember the key: HMOs are insurance companies, so they are most interested in the predictability of cost, for that will determine their medical loss exposure, which will in turn drive the premium that they need to charge in a very competitive market.

FIGURE 4–2

Revenue/Cost/Profit under Fee for Service

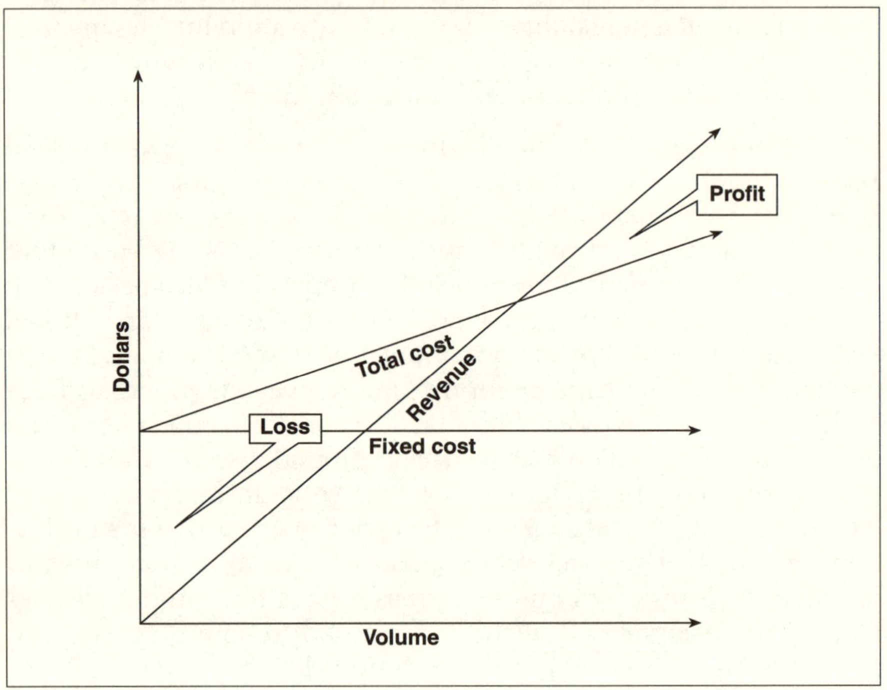

What are the critical success factors in MCO contracting?

- The ability to deliver services at a lower cost per unit, thereby earning a higher profit margin.
- The ability to deliver high quality service at a low cost per value, thereby getting the business from the plan.
- The ability to keep utilization at or below projections, thereby reducing consumption.
- The ability to care for larger numbers of patients.
- The ability to motivate and educate patients to be proactive.
- The ability to provide quality care with good outcomes.

In short, the ability to handle larger volumes of patients is one of the keys to capitation's success. Since you are being paid a fixed PMPM, a percentage of your overhead is being paid on a

FIGURE 4-3

Revenue/Cost/Profit under Capitation

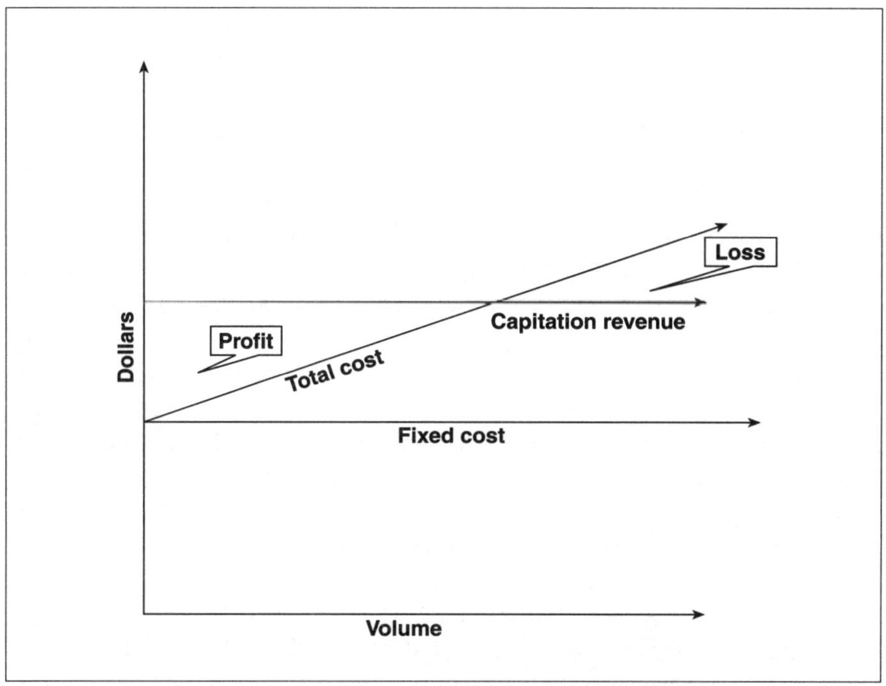

monthly basis by the health plan. The more patients assigned to the practice means more revenue to the practice. The more patients you can handle, then the lower the cost per unit of service. Yet the more services you render increases your total costs, and your profit margin declines. (In later pages we will discuss how to compute capitation and measure how it works.)

It is this inverse incentive that often confuses people and throws them astray. Under fee for service (FFS) or discounted FFS arrangements, the math is simple—more consumption of services leads to greater revenue and therefore greater profit.

Under capitation arrangements, however, this is reversed. Revenue also is fixed, and cost rises for each service provided. In effect, then, a practice begins with a profit margin in place. Since you already know what your revenue will be, you simply deduct the fixed costs and arrive at the beginning profit margin. Each time you serve a patient, there is the incremental or variable cost of that service—an expense that is a deduction from your beginning profit.

Earlier in this chapter, it was noted that capitation is a payment for standby costs, a retainer. Implicit in this arrangement is that you will be providing services. You do not expect to provide no services and keep all of the revenue as profit, any more than the life insurance company expects to keep all of the premium revenue and never pay death benefits. Your price—your capitation rate—needs to be sufficiently high to cover your costs of providing services and provide a profit margin for the physician owners.

On the other hand, there are negative aspects to capitation as well. First and foremost: you work more for less. The time, expense, and effort that go into treating and caring for a patient are not related directly to the fee earned. The key here is the average revenue yield, that is, the collected dollars for every hour of service. Simply comparing your full fee to the capitation rate or to a negotiated fee rate does not tell the true picture at all. A true measure is your collected dollars against what you have been effectively paid: charges less adjustments (uncollected, bad debt, contractual allowances, etc.).

MANAGEMENT STRATEGIES FOR CAPITATION

Under capitation you will have taken on the underwriting risk for providing a defined set of services for a defined set of patients, that is, a plan's covered lives. The task of the practice, then, is to manage its resources so that the practice can provide the services. As discussed above, the incentives and rewards under capitation are different and sometimes reversed from the incentives and rewards under fee for service. It almost reminds me of the mythical "antimatter parallel universe" of the "Star Trek" television show. In the parallel universe, everything is the same as the "original" universe that you and I live in, except it is reversed—good people are evil, and the like. Put the antimatter universe together with matter and KABOOM! End of both universes.

While it's not quite the same here, a collision of the two mindsets and strategies can lead to a management and organizational breakdown. For a capitated environment, there are three critical success factors:

1. The opportunities and negative aspects of capitation must be understood. Your revenue is predictable and steady, but the relationship between work effort, cost, and revenue is broken and changed.
2. Market share is key; your success will be determined in part by your ability to assume the responsibility and risk for caring for a larger patient population.
3. You will need to act like a traditional insurance company and undertake risk management and prevention activities as a long-term strategy to protect patients (assets) from illness and reduced activity (losses). Through prevention, utilization of more expensive services is reduced, thereby reducing the practice's costs and increasing its profits.

Capitation in Practice

In the real world, there are several management strategies in use to managing risk, including: (1) the gatekeeper physician; (2) subcapitation; and (3) the reverse gatekeeper (whereby specialists are capitated).

The use of a gatekeeper is the most common method used to control utilization of services. In a gatekeeper-based system, the role of the primary care physician (internist, family practitioner, obstetrician/gynecologist, or pediatrician) is to be the keeper of the gate, if you will, much like the green man guarding the gates to Oz. An HMO patient must go through the primary care physician to get referrals to virtually all specialties and other services. Absent the referral, the service doesn't get provided, or at least paid for, by the health care plan.

The gatekeeper has several roles:

- If the patient needs care, the gatekeeper does it or refers it.
- If a precertification is needed, the gatekeeper does it.
- If a consult is needed, the gatekeeper arranges for it.

- If a preauthorization is needed, the gatekeeper gets it.
- If a hospitalization is needed, the gatekeeper justifies it.

The paradox then for the gatekeeper, the primary care physician, is that he will spend less time with patients and more time on paperwork, phone calls, and follow up: that is, less time on direct patient care and more time managing care. The question he must present to himself then is, "Is all this worth it?" given the capitation rate he is being paid. Under managed care and capitation, the gatekeeper truly becomes a family physician responsible for the entire continuum of care. In addition to clinical skills, primary care physicians also require the full spectrum of patient management skills. This in turn may require more staff and more sophisticated computer systems; in short, the gatekeeper physician must possess the ability to track what is happening to his patients. From the patient's perspective, it could be very advantageous in that there is at least one person who knows or can readily know what is going on.

The gatekeeper system has come under increasing attack not so much because of the inherent function of approving referral, but rather due to the financial incentive built in to induce the physicians not to make a referral. These financial incentives can come in several forms, including:

- A referral fund pool where the physician and/or practice receives any funds in the PMPM set aside for specialty services that are not expended.
- A partial or full risk medical capitation arrangement, where the practice receives a PMPM and pays for specialty services out of the "global" PMPM paid by the HMO. Theoretically, the originating practice could spend down all of the PMPM funds in paying for specialty services and have no money left. (This is one place where stop loss arrangements become important.)
- Additions or subtractions from the practice's capitation rate based upon variance from budgeted specialty services utilized.

Incentives such as these put the PCP in a difficult position; PCPs are beginning, then, to ration health care. As the PMPM rates continue to edge downward in some markets, medical groups under full medical risk capitation are under increasing pressure to ration the use of specialty services (any service that will cause a flow of cash out of the practice) in order to pay overhead and a distribution to the owners.

So what are the practice's options for specialty care services? One option often used by groups in this situation is to do the same thing an HMO does—lock down the cost of specialty services. Just as the HMO has capitated the PCP group, so can the PCP group capitate the specialty services that it uses. This process is known as subcapitation and can go down several rungs of the health care food chain.

Let's use an example to show how subcapitation can work. Suppose:

Aaron's HMO pays full medical risk capitation PMPM to the PCP group:	$ 40/PMPM
Next, the PCP group contracts with several specialty groups for designated services, paying them a PMPM. The total cost is:	$ 20/PMPM
The PCP group remaining PMPM is:	$ 20/PMPM

Out of the amount remaining, the PCP will be responsible for paying claims for any professional services that are not under the capitation contract, such as when a patient chooses a specialty group that is in the HMO network, and therefore accessible to the patient, but for which the PCP has not contracted. As such, the PCP group must set up a reserve pool of funds, in much the same way as an insurance company does, to pay for claims.

Finally, since the PCP group is responsible for all professional service claims, it has a theoretically unlimited exposure to make cash outlays. To protect itself, the PCP group must have a stop loss plan. A stop loss plan is, as the name implies, an insurance policy with a high deductible. In the case of capitation plans, it typically will be designed to kick in when the expenses for a given case exceed a preset threshold. As an example, let's say the PCP group provides pediatric services itself. However, pediatric subspecialty services, such as neonatology, are on a fee-for-service basis. One year, there are two very sick premature babies born, and the professional fees reach $25,000 each, for a total of $50,000. The PCP group could have done two things to prevent such a high exposure: (1) entered into a subcapitation contract with the neonatal group, so that the neonatal group would have been paid a small PMPM for each covered life; or (2) taken out a stop loss policy. A stop loss policy is typically written on a per case basis. For example, when the professional fees in each of the above cases reached $5,000, any services above that point are paid out of the proceeds of the stop loss policy. The group's cash exposure, then, would not have been $50,000 for the two babies, but only $10,000.

Stop loss insurance itself comes in several forms, one through the HMO and the other which can be purchased through certain insurance carriers such as John Alden and Fortis. The policies usually are obtained through a broker, and the underwriting is specific to the group. Policies are usually written on a PMPM basis and some carriers have set a minimum premium of $5,000 per year. The insurer will look at such things as: the amount of risk assumed by the group; the ability of the group to manage and control utilization; and the experience of the group with these kinds of contracts. Underwriting is specific, then, to the group involved. If you are in a situation where you need to take out stop loss insurance, it is important and will be helpful to shop around.

Following is an example of the initial questionnaire that is used by excess carriers. It is presented to give you a feel for the kinds of information that are requested.

The other way that stop loss insurance is purchased is through the HMO. The HMO may simply assume some or all of the additional risk or place part of the risk through its own stop loss insurance, or reinsurance. Here, too, the stop loss plan will be on a PMPM basis. In much the same way that you can save money on an auto policy by taking a higher deductible, the cost of a stop loss plan, as reflected in a deduction from your PMPM,

FIGURE 4-4

Physician Excess Stop Loss Questionnaire (Sample)

Name of Organization: ______________________________

Address: ______________________________

____

Type of Practice:

_____ Primary care _____ Specialty care (specify: ______________)

_____ Multispecialty:

List specialties: ______________________________

	Capitated Members				
HMOs covered	**Current**	**In 1 Yr.**	**Commercial**	**Medicare**	**Medicaid**

Are there any services that your group is not able to provide, but for which you are responsible under the terms of your contract? Please describe below:

Type of Service: **Designated group or facility** **Discounts/special rates in place? Describe**

____

____

____

____

What approximate percentage of services are delivered by:

Affiliated or in-network providers? _____ % Unaffiliated providers? _____ %

Please provide the details of contracts with affiliated providers.

Date you would like coverage to take effect: __________

Definition of eligible charges:

( ) ______ Fee schedule

RVU unit values (if applicable) ______ (please provide)

( ) % of billed charges

Coinsurance % that must be met: ______________________

Continued

FIGURE 4–4 Continued

Claims Experience:

List past three years' claims experience for all patients whose charges exceeded requested deductible. Include:

- Membership per year
- Dates of service
- Dates of birth
- Reason for services
- Total amount of charges billed
- Payment basis (FFS, discount, capitation)
- Amount recovered from reinsurance

List all current patients who would be covered under this policy who are potential reinsurance claimants.

Note: Determine number of active patients (any patient seen in past two years)

will vary depending upon the threshold where the stop loss kicks in. For example, with a $5,000 stop loss threshold, the full medical risk PMPM might be $30. With a $20,000 threshold, however, your PMPM might be $31.50. With the higher threshold you might be getting paid a higher PMPM. However, you have assumed more risk, so if patients incur the higher expenses, you are responsible for more of their care costs until the stop loss threshold is passed.

A stop loss plan also can be effectuated through the use of "risk bands." Risk bands are sometimes an intermediate step toward full risk capitation. Although using capitation, services rendered above the threshold are paid for on a fee-for-service basis. Risk bands also can be used on a "gross" basis; that is, it is not important how much is spent in services on an individual case, what matters is what the HMO expends overall for a group in a year's time.

Under a risk band scenario, a primary care group is to be paid a PMPM by the HMO. It receives the PMPM every month, as always. However, since this is a new contract, there is "pent up" demand for primary care services, so it is anticipated that patients

FIGURE 4–5

Capitation Risk Bands

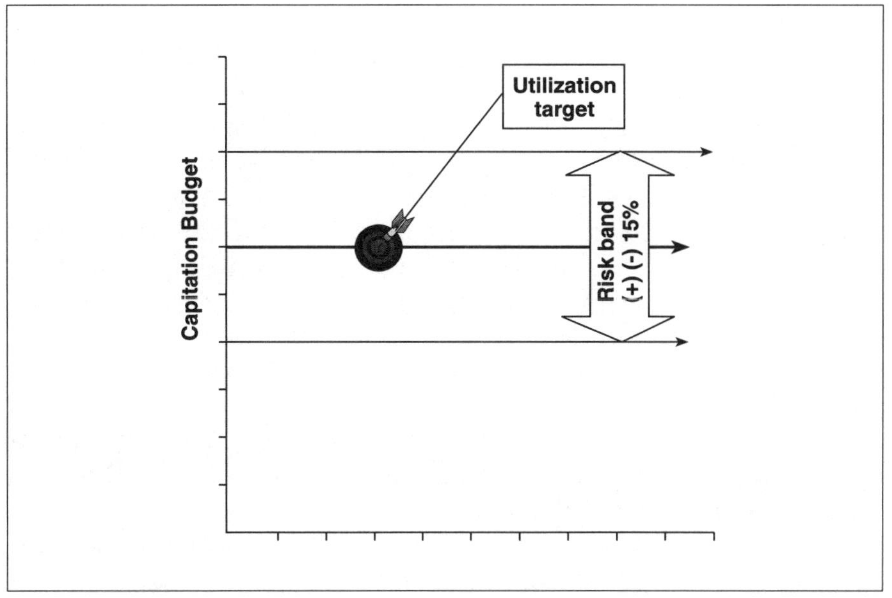

will be coming to the group at a higher rate than would otherwise be projected. Since the group has no experience in managing demand for PCP services, much less for specialty services, the HMO agrees to offer stop loss coverage.

The key elements to a risk band plan are: (1) determining the threshold; and (2) determining the fee schedule. Using the HMO's actuarial projections (and/or your own), you can establish a projected utilization of services. Since the capitation rate has been negotiated, you already know your estimated revenue for the year. As you provide services in the course of the year, the practice will bill the HMO, recording the fees incurred on a fee-for-service basis. When the fees incurred exceed the threshold amount, the practice will be paid additional monies on a fee-for-service basis. The additional amount might be a set fee schedule, usual and customary reimbursement (UCR) based fees, or a discount from the practice's full fee schedule. In either event, the HMO is paying additional monies to the practice above the capitation rate.

The assumption behind a risk band is that the projected utilization and expense is a forecast and will not be perfect. Within a range plus or minus from the target point, only the capitation rate will be paid. A range of plus or minus 15 percent is a wide range—a group new to this would be more conservative and would look for a band with a range of plus or minus 2 to 3 percent. The band can then be widened each year, thereby assuming more risk each time. If billed fees exceed the "ceiling" (top line) of the band, the practice receives extra monies. If actual utilization is below the "basement" (lower line) of the band, the practice may be allowed to keep the full capitation amount. In that scenario, the utilization target may then be lowered the following year, as the practice has demonstrated that it can manage care and utilization of services. In some instances, such as a contract I once negotiated, the HMO receives a rebate if the actual utilization is below the basement line. The HMO receives a portion of the difference between the basement line and the actual utilization; this rebate is offered in recognition that the HMO has some role in lowering utilization.

Since the risk band system may require a fee schedule to work, you may be asking yourself, "We spend months negotiating the contract and a capitation rate, and now we need to come up with a fee schedule?!" Yes, you do, or you can use relative value units (RVUs) and back into a conversion factor and then into a fee schedule.

The main interest of an HMO is to establish predictability in its medical costs. You, on the other hand, need some protection in the event that utilization far exceeds projections, particularly if there are fluctuation risks that come into play and are beyond your control.

An easy way to come up with a fee schedule is presented in Table 4–1 (page 104). Your objective here is to use the RVU system to generate a fee schedule, relying upon the common acceptance of the RVU system. The underlying assumption behind RVUs is that, relative to each other, the units account for the variances in practice expense and work effort. If you recall when the RVU system was first introduced in 1992 by Medicare and imposed nationally, the idea was to equalize the basis for payment and reimbursement between specialists and primary care physicians. There have been various systems around but Medicare, through HCFA, chose to contract with a group from Harvard University to develop and modify a system. The argument historically had been that those physicians who do a "thing" (procedures such as surgery and testing) are paid much more than the "thinking" specialties in the primary care arena. As a result, there was an economic incentive, and not necessarily one good for patients, that rewarded physicians when treating patients using procedures and doing a "thing" as opposed to using less invasive and less costly measures.

RVUs consist of three components: (1) practice work effort; (2) practice expense; and (3) malpractice expense. These three components each have a number that has been derived based upon a sampling of practices throughout the country and the input from many of the medical specialty societies. By adding up the values of each of the three components, a number value is then derived for each CPT code. To account for the cost of living, particularly labor, in the various market areas around the country, the number is then adjusted by a geographic adjustment factor (GAF). There is a different GAF for each market area. The market GAF is then multiplied against the RVU for each component of each CPT code to determine the RVU for each code. This process is done for each and every code. Fortunately, your Medicare intermediary should provide you with the updated values each year.

Medicare reimbursement is driven by where the location of the practice is, not the residence of the patient. If a practice, however, has more than one office, it is very possible that it will receive different reimbursements, depending upon the office. The idea behind all these systems was to impose market discipline and market forces into health care. Despite a great degree of uncertainty, misunderstanding, and lack of information on the part of the HCFA, the system as used by Medicare has achieved fairly wide acceptance and is being utilized for a variety of management measures.

To use RVUs to develop a fee schedule, two key assumptions have to be made:

1. The average number of covered lives under the capitation contract.
2. The utilization by CPT code for the MCO's patients.

By working with the MCO itself, a practice can develop an assumption that both parties agree to as to the average number of covered lives per month that the practice will be responsible for in the coming contract year.

To develop a projected utilization by code, the practice can hire an actuary to make these projections. Yet, given the level of detail and the often small numbers involved, developing a projected utilization on a CPT code level is difficult and subject to a high error rate.

Another way to accomplish this involves establishing a conversion factor (CF) for relative value units (RVUs). By using a conversion factor, you then determine a fee schedule without any further discussion, using the same methodology as used by Medicare.

In order to "sell" this methodology to an MCO, you need to determine a conversion factor that will arrive at a "budget neutral" position; that is, regardless of whether paid on a capitation rate based upon a projected utilization of services or paid on a discounted fee-for-service basis, the MCO will pay the practice the same amount of money either way.

The steps to accomplish this are as follows:

1. Compute the capitation revenue:
   a. Determine the average number of covered lives per month.
   b. Multiply the average number of covered lives per month by the PMPM.
   c. Add the estimated copayments and coinsurance.
   d. Compute total capitation revenue.
2. Develop a utilization rate by CPT code:
   a. Determine the total number of active patients in your practice.
   b. Determine the utilization by CPT code.
   c. For each CPT code, determine the rate of utilization per 1,000 patients by dividing the utilization by the total number of active patients (for example: 150 services in a patient base of 10,000 = a rate of 15 per 1,000 patients).
3. Determine the projected utilization per CPT code. For each CPT code, apply the utilization rate per 1,000 patients to the estimated average number of covered lives to determine the projected utilization by CPT code for the MCO's patients.

4. Determine the total projected number of RVUs to be provided in the year:
   a. For each CPT code, multiply the projected utilization of services by the RVU for the code to determine the total projected number of RVUs to be delivered in the year.
   b. Add all of the totals derived in step 4.*a* for all of the CPT codes to determine the total projected number of RVUs to be delivered in the year.
5. Divide the total projected dollars to be paid under capitation by the total projected number of RVUs to determine a conversion factor.
6. Multiply the conversion factor by the RVU for each CPT code to determine a "fee" for each code.

Tables 4–1 and 4–2 present the procedure described above. A note about common procedure terminology (CPT) codes should be mentioned here.* CPT codes have been developed and are managed by the American Medical Association, which updates the codes every year. It is important that you obtain the updated code books from one of the publishers (there are several) which are typically available in the fall, to check to see if there have been changes in the coding for services that you provide. Very often, state and specialty medical societies will alert you of any major changes pending. It is important that you code to the fullest degree, not so much as a means of unbundling services but more importantly because more refined subcodes may exist that will be more descriptive of the services rendered. There are bundling and unbundling issues that you will need to deal with on an individual basis. The key objective is to fairly represent what you have done.

As you can see, there are many variations on the theme that you may be presented with or that you can propose yourself. Always remember the key principles, however, and protect yourself.

As noted earlier, capitation has its good points and its bad points. Under capitation there are a number of opportunities. First and foremost you are assured a steady, predictable cash flow. It is much like a retainer. Under capitation one of the big advantages is

---

*CPT codes are a copyright of the American Medical Association, Chicago, IL.

TABLE 4–1

Calculating a Conversion Factor from the PMPM

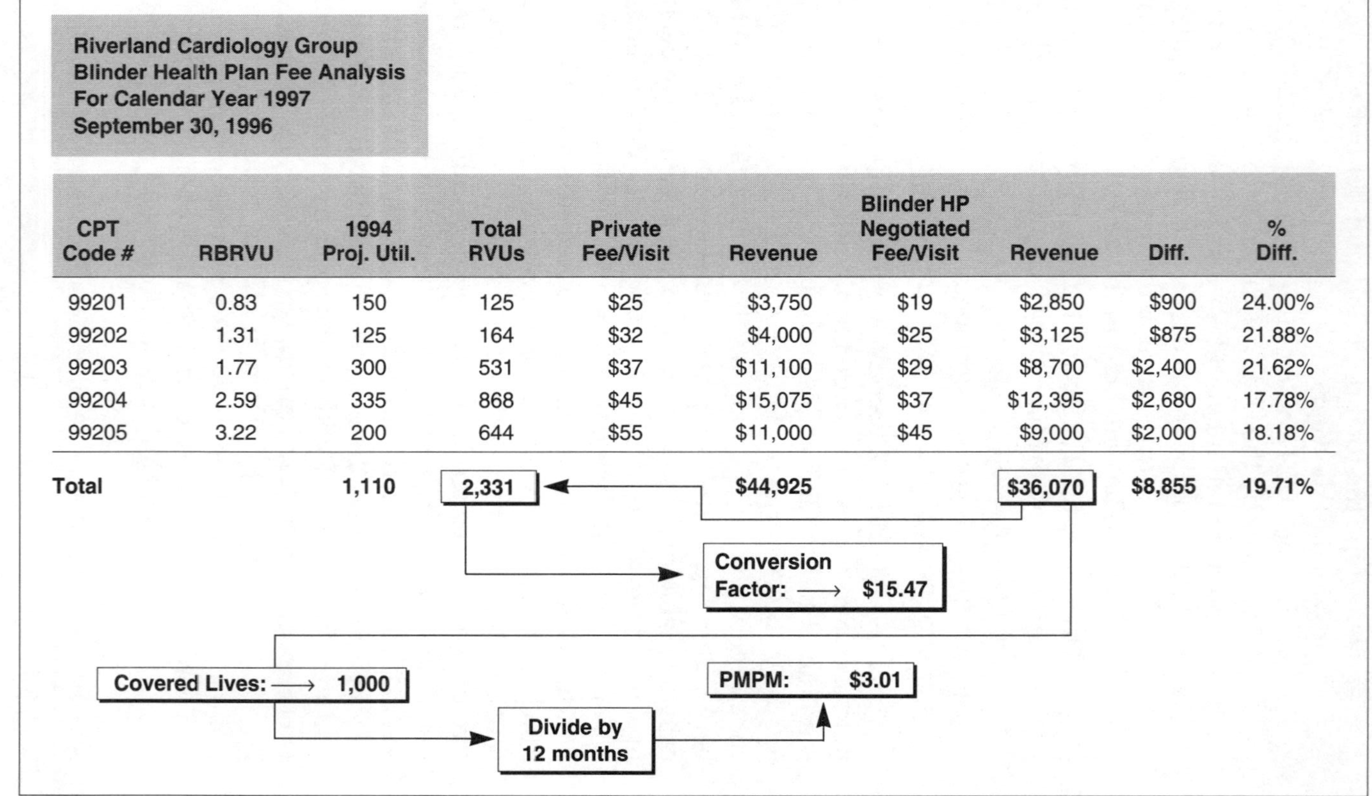

Riverland Cardiology Group
Blinder Health Plan Fee Analysis
For Calendar Year 1997
September 30, 1996

CPT Code #	RBRVU	1994 Proj. Util.	Total RVUs	Private Fee/Visit	Revenue	Blinder HP Negotiated Fee/Visit	Revenue	Diff.	% Diff.
99201	0.83	150	125	$25	$3,750	$19	$2,850	$900	24.00%
99202	1.31	125	164	$32	$4,000	$25	$3,125	$875	21.88%
99203	1.77	300	531	$37	$11,100	$29	$8,700	$2,400	21.62%
99204	2.59	335	868	$45	$15,075	$37	$12,395	$2,680	17.78%
99205	3.22	200	644	$55	$11,000	$45	$9,000	$2,000	18.18%
Total		**1,110**	**2,331**		**$44,925**		**$36,070**	**$8,855**	**19.71%**

Conversion Factor: ⟶ $15.47
Covered Lives: ⟶ 1,000
Divide by 12 months
PMPM: $3.01

TABLE 4–2

Applying a Conversion Factor to a Fee

Riverland Cardiology Group
Blinder H.P. Capitation Fee Analysis
For Calendar Year 1997
September 30, 1996

CPT Code #	RVUs	1994 Proj. Util.	Total RVUs	Private Fee	Revenue	Conversion Rate	Blinder HP Fee/Visit	Revenue	Diff.	% Diff.
99201	0.83	150	125	$25	$3,750	$15.47	$13	$1,926	$12	48.64%
99202	1.31	125	164	$32	$4,000	$15.47	$20	$2,533	$12	36.67%
99203	1.77	300	531	$37	$11,100	$15.47	$27	$8,215	$10	25.99%
99204	2.59	335	868	$45	$15,075	$15.47	$40	$13,423	$5	10.96%
99205	3.22	200	644	$55	$11,000	$15.47	$50	$9,963	$5	9.43%
Total		**1,110**	**2,331**		**$44,925**			**$36,059**	$8,866	19.74%

RVU × Conversion Rate = Fee

that your bad debt burden is reduced if not eliminated. The practice is paid the PMPM on a monthly basis, but you are responsible for collecting the copayment at the time of service. This is a point that cannot be overemphasized. It is the responsibility of the provider to collect the copayment. Under the terms of the policy, it is the clear responsibility of the patient to pay this fee at the time of service. You do not want to be faced with having to bill for a $10, and sometimes a $2, copayment fee.

Another opportunity of capitation is that you are rewarded for being a better manager. Your revenue is essentially fixed, and cash flow is predictable. Capitation is likely to be only a portion of your revenue for a year. The balance will come from various fee-for-service plans, including Medicare. Capitation is much like the social security check in a person's retirement income, it represents the "fixed income" portion, versus the "flexible" income that comes from private pension plans and savings. The good news is that a portion of your income is assured, the bad news is that the expenses related to that income are neither fixed nor completely controllable.

Computing Capitation

As you can see, capitation is actually a very simple concept: you as a provider get paid a fixed amount of money every month to be responsible for the care of a given set of people.

Here again, we turn to the question: are we making or losing money? One way to assess the answer is to compare the revenue from a capitation contract to what the revenue would have been if fee-for-service was being billed. Table 4–3 presents the formula used to make this comparison.

There is, however, a caveat about this worksheet: it only works for primary care practices. The critical assumption in this formula is that the rate of utilization of services is similar between fee-for-services and HMO patients. The formula is based upon developing a rate of utilization of the practice's services among the current patient base, and applying that utilization rate to the HMO population. A person may identify themselves as a patient of a primary care practice simply by seeing the physician once, or as a result of enrolling in an HMO. The primary care practice, then, has an identifiable core of patients, who may or may not utilize their services.

TABLE 4–3

Capitation Fee Analysis

Riverland Primary
Blinder H.P. Capitation Fee Analysis
For Calendar Year 1996

CPT Code #	RVUs	1995 Total Utilization	Utilization Rate Per 1,000 Patients	Blinder H.P. Projected Utilization	Private Fee	Projected Revenue	Capitation Rate	Difference
99201	0.83	150	15.00	19	$25	$475	$.50 PMPM	
99202	1.31	125	12.50	16	$32	$512	× 1250 covered lives =	
99203	1.77	300	30.00	38	$37	$1,406	$625	
99204	2.59	335	33.50	42	$45	$1,890	× 12 =	
99205	3.22	200	20.00	25	$55	$1,375	+ copays ($750)	
Total		**1,110**	**111.00**	**139**		**$5,658**		
					Collection rate	**80%**		
					Net Cash Revenue:	**$4,526**	**$8,250** →	**$2,592**

Assumptions:

1. 10,000 Patients in practice base
2. 1,250 covered lives assigned to Riverland Primary Care

Formulas:

1. Take total utilization by CPT code and determine rate per 1,000 (or 100) patients. The result is column 4.
2. Multiply column 4 by number of covered lives; this equals the projected utilization for members (column 5).
3. Multiply column 5 by fee-for-service, then adjust by collection rate to get projected revenue under a FFS arrangement.
4. Calculate capitation revenue: PMPM multiplied by number of covered lives multiplied by 12 months = total revenue. Add all copayments.
5. Compare net cash collections with capitation income.

When an HMO signs a contract with a practice, the HMO will identify a group of "patients" who are assigned to the practice and may or may not seek services. Specialists, however, have a different relationship with their patients. By and large, people are "patients" of a specialty practice on an episodic basis. People become patients when there is a need for the specialist's services, and once a course of treatment is completed or embarked on, the relationship often ends. In summary, a utilization rate of a PCP's patient base can be applied against the patient base supplied by an HMO. A utilization rate for specialty services only tells a practice what will be the potential utilization of services once a member has been referred and becomes a patient. This may be important information, but it does not answer the critical question: given a certain population group, how many and what kinds of services will a specialist be called upon to provide? Later in this chapter we will discuss some other means of assessing the capitation rate. To assess the capitation rate, prepare a list of all your CPT codes or a sampling of your major CPT codes. As Table 4–3 shows, enter the RVU for each CPT code, the number of services delivered by code in the last year, and your current private pay (gross) fee. An underlying assumption, and a proper one in computing capitation income, is that the age and acuity distribution of your current patient base should approximate what a new HMO, without any history with you, should provide to you. There is anecdotal evidence to suggest that this is in fact what happens, and it makes a certain amount of intuitive sense. One of the due diligence checks you make in assessing a managed care contract is investigating whether the managed care plan is going out and seeking higher risk members than you have typically been seeing. But assuming that is not the case, let's continue this scenario and you will see how it works.

Your next step is to multiply the charges by actual utilization to get your current gross charges. Add all these charges up and you will have your total charges for the year. Then adjust by multiplying your full charges by your actual collection rate. This collection is the percentage of full charges that you actually collect in cash. Using this collection rate, you then would account for all contractual allowances, discounts, write-offs, and such. From that number, which is your actual collections, you can now take your net charges, divide by the number of individual patients you have treated, and arrive at your revenue per year. Divide that number by 12 and you have the per month for each patient, which is the equivalent of the PMPM. You may find that your PMPM in real life may even be higher than an offer by an HMO. At the very least, you now have a firm basis from which to make a comparison.

A specialty physician practice could consider using a slightly different comparison. Rather than calculating the net HMO revenue per month on a PMPM basis, instead consider calculating the net revenue per HMO patient per month. To do this, take the net HMO revenue for a month (the right side of Table 4-3) and divide this number by the number of individual patients from the HMO who were treated that month. The result (the quotient) is the HMO Revenue Per Patient Per Month. Compare that number to the Non-HMO Revenue Per Patient Per Month, and the practice has numbers to compare.

Both methods presented above are founded upon the assumption that the rate of utilization of services will be the same for HMO patients and non-HMO patients. There is anecdotal experience to suggest that utilization will increase for primary care services. Since these calculations are based upon historical data and are forecasts of future activity, they will be wrong. After the first pass is made for these calculations, run the numbers again by changing the utilization rate: assume that the HMO population will utilize services 5 percent, 10 percent, 20 percent, and so on, higher than the non-HMO data. You can then plug these numbers into the profit and loss projections for a practice and see what impact varying utilization rates and capitation rates will have on a practice's revenue and profitability.

Another method of evaluating the PMPM capitation rate is based on your practice expenses. The underlying assumption here is that the payer does not materially affect the cost of caring for a patient in like circumstances and presentation. That being the case, in order to evaluate a proposed PMPM capitation rate, it is necessary to know what your costs are on a per patient basis.

In order to compute the practice's cost per patient, simply take all the costs of the practice and divide by 12, for the total cost per month. You will then divide the total practice cost per month by the number of active patients in your practice. I define active patients as any patient that the practice has seen in the past two years. I also in-

TABLE 4–4

Computing Practice Cost Per Patient Per Month

Personnel:	
Salaries	
Benefits	Staff cost PPPM
Nonpersonnel Expenses:	
Occupancy	
Rent/depreciation	
Utilities	
Maintenance	
Supplies	
Other overhead	Overhead cost PPPM
	= Total PPPM cost
	+ Profit margin
	= Total price PPPM

Cost divided by number of patients (members) divided by 12 = Cost PPPM (Per Patient Per Month)

clude employee (nonpartner or nonshareholder) salaries and benefits as practice expenses. Those physicians who are owners of a practice, either partners or shareholders, do not truly draw a salary. Owners are ultimately at risk for meeting the obligations of the practice, so that any monies that they can take out of the practice are really profit. Even if the owners draw checks at the same time as payroll, and even if they process the checks through the payroll system, the checks represent an advance on profit distribution.

Table 4–4 presents how the Practice Cost Per Patient Per Month is developed.

Now that the Practice Cost Per Patient Per Month (PPPM) has been computed, it needs to be compared to something. Comparing it to the PMPM rate doesn't work because the practice is being paid for the HMO's members who will never use the physicians. Instead, the same comparison as used for specialists to assess their capitation rate is used: compare the Practice Cost PPPM to the HMO Revenue PPPM. The calculation is as follows:

1. Calculate the total revenue from the one HMO that Month. Include capitation payments, copayments, and such.
2. Divide the total revenue by the number of individual patients who sought services, regardless of the number or types of services rendered.

The difference between the Practice Cost PPPM is the profit margin for the practice.

Running these calculations for your practice are each critical pieces of information that, together with the Due Diligence Checklist and other research on your part, come together to build the portrait of the HMO. Then, and only then, do you have the information to make the management judgments necessary to negotiate and execute the best possible contract with an HMO or other managed care organization.

Capitation is a payment system that imposes significant new responsibilities and risks on physicians and medical practices. Nevertheless, you still can maintain a viable, reasonably healthy practice by adhering to certain principles:

1. Read and understand the contract.
2. Compute the cost of providing your services (see Chapter 7).
3. Bill promptly, electronically, and follow up often.
4. Collect copayments at time of service.
5. Run a patient-focused practice.
6. Train your staff and invest in its education.
7. Teach patients about health and their health plan.
8. Market yourself—build and maintain relationships with the other physicians and the business community.
9. Be vigilant about the quality and utilization of services.
10. Grow bigger and take on more covered lives.

5 CHAPTER

Focus on Operations

Many things change when you sign a contract with a managed care plan. Almost everyone talks about the changes in your reimbursement, particularly when you are capitate (see Chapter 4). What trips up many practices, however, are the operational implications of the contract. Remember that, unlike indemnity plans, the practice now has a contractual relationship with the carrier, and implicit within the notion of a contract is that each party has a set of responsibilities to the other party. In this chapter, we will walk through a typical patient office visit, discussing where and how operational procedures need to be changed both to comply with contractual requirements and to be best organized to succeed with these contracts.

An office visit is much more than the time spent in an exam room with a physician. There are a number of steps and numerous personal and system interactions that take place between the practice and the practice staff and the patient. Forms need to be completed, medical record charts pulled and delivered on the right day to the right person, the bill filed with the right insurance company on the right form and sent the proper way to the right location, and so on.

The following flowchart presents, on a simplified scale, the flow of the patients and the paper connected with a simple office visit.

FIGURE 5–1

Patient Paper Flow

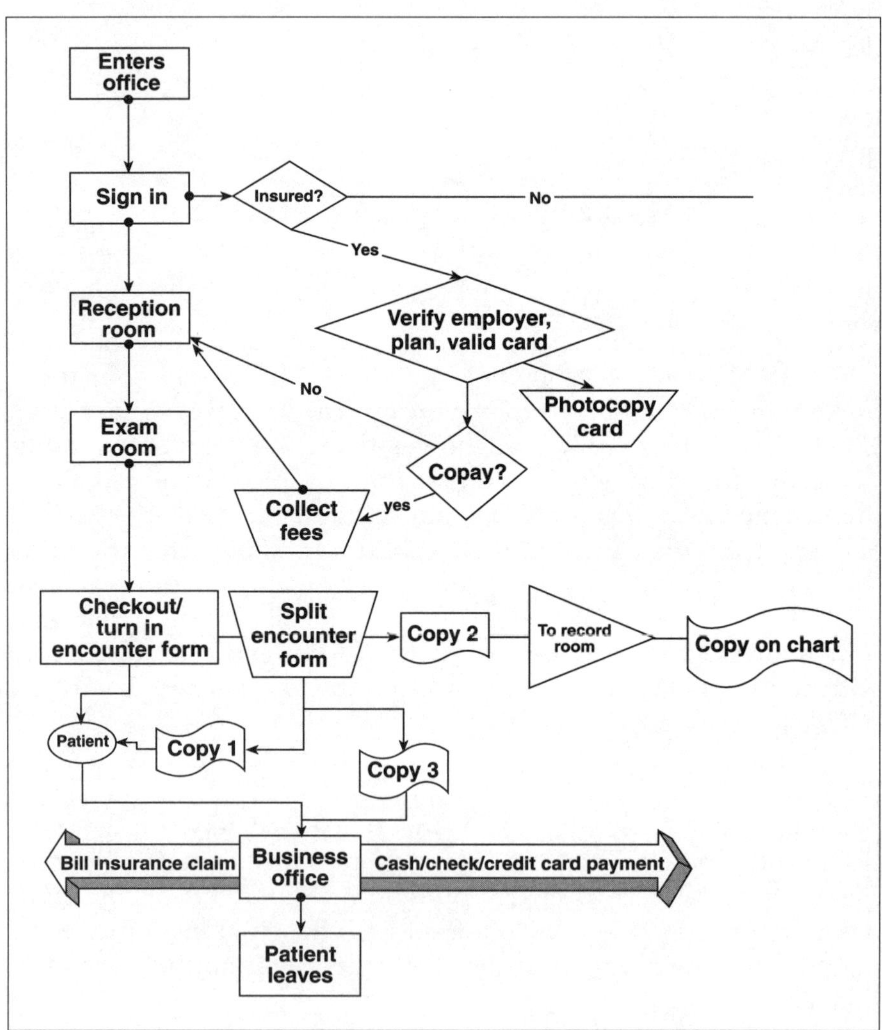

THE APPOINTMENT DESK

The "window to the world," if you will, in a physician's practice is the appointment desk. For patients, this is the point of entry into the practice. The schedule used by the practice is managed by the appointment desk, which determines how many patients can be seen, by whom, and in which location on a given day. The appointment desk can hustle and be creative and help a patient to be seen despite a crowded schedule, or it can go the easy route and mindlessly follow the options put forward by the scheduling software. It can request an additional slot to add another patient in, or it can passively just tell the patient, "Sorry, our next appointment is in two months."

Try calling your office sometime and see how you are treated. I was once on a consulting project for a hospital, and there was disagreement within the community as to whether there were enough physicians. One of my tasks was to call a dozen members of the medical staff, pretend that I was a new patient, and see how soon I could be seen. My report back to the client was that I could easily be seen that same day, or the next day at the latest. Every office also suggested that I could go to the emergency room (fortunately suggesting the client's ER!). I had to think fast on my feet, because each office asked me a series of questions about my symptoms in order to provide better information to the physician, and each was ready to schedule an appointment on the spot! I was rather impressed and could safely tell the hospital that a physician shortage did not appear to be its problem.

THE TELEPHONE

For a practice, the telephones are the principal instrument of communication. Information is the lifeblood of a practice, everything from clinical information about patients to business information concerning the management of the practice.

The way in which the phones are answered conveys an immediate and powerful image to the caller as to the kind of organization it is. Compare, for example, the following telephone greetings:

- "Doctor's office."
- "Drs. Jones, Smith, and Steel. This is Mary. How may I help you?"

- "Great Doctors, how may I direct your call?"
- "Great Doctors, please hold." (click—dead air)

When the phone is answered, that moment is a deciding one for the patient—Am I of importance to the practice? Answering with the practice's name confirms that the caller has reached the right office. Giving a name and saying, "How may I help you?" is a friendly greeting. A truly busy practice may delete the personal identification when someone is in a phone operator position, simply answering the main number and transferring the call. When that is done, however, the following two critical procedures must be in place.

1. In transferring, there cannot be any dead space while one holds; the caller won't be able to tell if he has been disconnected. To prevent this from happening, you can add an "on-hold" tape system, which will cut on when the person is put on hold. This can be music, or a more appropriate tape that is a recording of health-related and practice-related messages, such as:

> The office hours for Great Doctors are 8 AM to 5 PM, Monday through Friday. At all other times, one of our physicians is on call and available to help our patients. Always call our office number to reach a Great Doctors . . . Did you know that walking is one of the best and most popular forms of exercise? A brisk 20 minute walk three times a week can make a difference in how you feel and in your overall health . . . The flu shot is available now—please schedule an appointment with our nurse during this phone call. . . . (Then repeat.)

As a rule, a caller should not hear the message repeated, which means that all calls should be answered by a live person within 20 seconds at most. (If you think this is too short a time, try waiting on hold for that long yourself.) To be safe, a two minute tape should be made. These are special tapes known as "continuous loop." They can be recorded on a regular machine. You might employ a small local radio station to make the tape for you, using the voice of one of the physicians or the station's talent. Such a recording can be done for as little as $100 in some areas, and a "professional" recording will sound better to callers.

2. When the call is answered, the staff person should again identify her area and name, as in "Appointment Desk, this is Mary

Jones, how may I help you?" This confirms for the caller that they have been transferred to the right area and that someone is ready to help them.

A transferred call should also be answered within three to five rings. If more than five rings, the call should automatically ring back to the reception desk. The reception desk should take a message, a phone number, and give the call the highest priority so that it is returned within 1 hour for patient calls, and within 24 hours for other business calls.

By the nature of their work, physicians often cannot take a call when it comes in. During office hours, priority must be given to patients who have appointments as opposed to callers. Have you ever been in a store and the clerk takes a phone call and spends time with that customer rather than you, who are standing before them? Too many practices, however, then just stack up messages with those famous parting words to the patient, "The doctor will get back to you." So, the patient waits . . . and waits . . . never knowing when the returned call will come.

Phones are an integral part of the practice of medicine in the 1990s, as computers will be in the next century. Since patient calls are part of the practice, book time during the day—perhaps every hour—to return these calls. Trying to squeeze them in between patients simply doesn't work; calls may not get made until the end of the day, by which time the patient may have gotten tired of waiting and left. Or, the reception room may start to fill up as you fall behind in your schedule.

When a patient calls for an appointment, it is important that the staff verify certain financial information. A patient's insurance coverage now has an impact on medical decision making—what procedures can be used, what prescriptions will be covered (and at what out-of-pocket cost to the patient), and who can provide care. When the appointment call comes in to a specialist's office, the staff must verify that a referral has been approved by the patient's primary care physician (PCP). Some managed care organizations (MCOs) require that all referrals for specialty services be called in and that a referral number or other tracking method be generated. The specialist's office will need to know this information before proceeding.

In addition, the staff should verify or collect the following information for new patients:

- Patient's name.
- Name of insured (or responsible party).
- Address.
- Phone (home and work). Do you expect to be at work the day before or the day of the appointment? This question is asked so that you can actually reach the patient if you need to. I have often come home to a blinking light on my answering machine with a physician's office trying to reach me.
- Employer (of patient and insured).
- Name of insurance plan, group name, and all numbers (remember, there may be a suffix if the patient is a dependent, and the dependent can be either spouse!).

The appointment desk also serves as the screening and diversion point of the practice. Managed care plans place high premiums on controlling the utilization of services, but the foundation of that critical factor is that preventative medical care given by the primary care physician is the optimal way to achieve that goal, particularly when looking at a long time horizon. Under indemnity plans, the incentive was to see any patient who wanted to see you. Under a capitated contract, you only want to see those patients who need to see you. An example of this occurs during the flu season, when for many patients, there is nothing you can do for them. While living in Pittsburgh, I was a member of a staff model health maintenance organization (HMO). One winter, I had a very bad cold and called my internist. I was immediately transferred to the phone nurses, who asked me a series of questions and then concluded the call by telling me that the symptoms I described were going around, that the only thing that could be done was aspirin and hot liquids, and to call if there was a marked change. There wasn't a chance I was going to see a physician, but then again, did I need to see one if there was nothing he could do for me anyhow?

Each practice needs to decide what it is comfortable with, but in essence, the focus of the appointment desk is to best schedule the physicians' time for the patients who need to see and be examined by a physician, as opposed to those who they *think* need to see one.

Much of the flow of calls into an office is of a routine nature. Prescription refills are a common occurrence, as are calls with billing questions. Rather than tying up your incoming patient lines with calls that will only be transferred, dedicate several of your lines for specific purposes, such as (1) prescription refills; (2) business office questions; and (3) "personal calls" for physicians and staff.

Telephone bills, while sometimes annoyingly high, really constitute a small part of the practice expense. The telephone is the "face" of the practice to the outside world. When a patient, or prospective patient, calls a practice for the first time, the manner in which the phone is answered sets a tone for the relationship.

A note about voice prompt systems that answer the phone and instruct you through a menu of choices. Before installing such a system, include the option to hit "0" to go directly to a receptionist. Patients from the older generations are less likely to like these systems, so you also must consider carefully how your patients will respond to the system.

The telephone remains the principal means of communication for a physician practice. To be effective, the phones must be answered promptly and the call dispatched to the proper person with a minimum of delay. As technology advances and computers and telephones merge, the capabilities of phone systems continue to grow. Automatic attendant, voice mail, remote access, "fax back," and one number calling, are just some of the capabilities that a practice can put to use.

Your phone system, then, is critical to the operation of the practice. The task for the phone system is to be able to answer, screen, and route phone calls. The system also can be used to receive and convey information.

This same modern technology can put people on interminable hold or drop them into "voice mail hell." Much like the man named Charlie on the MTA (the man who never returned) callers can get into some phone systems and never get out. Your system, then, needs to be easy to use, possess simple, clear instructions, and always have an escape.

First and foremost, all calls are to be answered promptly—within three rings. If a live person cannot answer, the system should have the capability to answer the call using an "automated attendant." You're probably familiar with these systems, in which a soothing voice reassures the caller, "One of our courteous operators will be with you shortly." After this "answer," however, many of the systems leave the caller with "dead" air—complete silence, interrupted perhaps by an occasional click or other sound. Many organizations have found, then, that the caller becomes confused and uncertain as to whether or not the call is still connected.

Two points about placing callers on hold: this time should be kept to a minimum, but while you have someone on hold, put the time to good use. As mentioned above, as a general rule, a caller should not be on hold for more than 20 seconds. If that sounds like a short period of time, sit down and time out 20 seconds, and you will see that it seems like a very long time to a caller. The second rule is that a person should not be transferred more than once without one of the practice's staff taking responsibility for handling the call. For example: a call is answered by the receptionist, and the caller asks to speak to a medical assistant. The caller explains her question, and the medical assistant is not sure where to transfer the call but thinks she knows who can help the caller. Before transferring the call, the assistant should make sure that the caller has the extension and name of the person to whom they are being transferred, in the event that the call is disconnected. Better yet, if the staff person isn't sure, then she should take the caller's name and phone number and take responsibility for finding out who can help this caller. Once the staff person has found this information she will need to convey the caller's information to the right person and let that person call the patient back; doing this completes the loop—the original staff person has made the "proper" referral, and the original caller knows that her call has been handled and that she will get a call back.

Back to being on hold: we've all been in the situation where the call is answered, transferred, and we are on hold. Or the automatic attendant answers the call and then puts us on hold while we await the outcome. Put this time to good use. Now, we've all laughed at the companies that place advertisements anywhere people stop for two seconds—the front of shopping carts, television monitors above the supermarket checkout line, restroom stalls, and so on. In fact, this makes good business sense. While your callers are on hold, you can be playing the "on-hold" tape discussed earlier in this chapter. These messages need to be short because people should not be on hold for a long period of time. I was negotiating a contract with an HMO once, and I was, of course, on hold while my call to the administrator was being transferred. On came the tape with health education snippets. I once asked the administrator to be put back on hold so that I could hear the rest of the information!

The goal of telephone management is to ease access as well as offload phone traffic from a central receptionist, who may have multiple duties. Having telephone lines dedicated to appointments, business office, prescription refills, and general/all other generally will cover the key areas. To accomplish this, you need to develop a phone plan, which is not a difficult exercise. The objective of the phone plan is to document the types of calls your practice receives, their potential destination points, and procedures for handling the common types of calls.

The first step, then, is to develop the telephone triage table (see Table 5–1). This plan contains the following information:

- Destination points for calls. This includes any extension where a staff person will answer a call.
- Issue responsibility. What "types" of calls (what subject) are assigned to which person or persons. This helps to insure that there is clear responsibility assigned for likely issues that will be raised by callers.

The next step is to assess the call volume within your own practice and allocate lines from there. To accomplish this, have the reception desk staff maintain a phone log for a few weeks. For each call coming in, a checkoff should be made as to where the call has been transferred. This should be done in one-hour blocks of time, as shown in the call transfer log (Table 5–2).

TABLE 5-1

Telephone Triage Plan

Location (destination points for incoming calls)	Extension/Direct Dial Number	Issue Responsibilities
Reception	1234	
Administration	1235	Practice information
Administrator	1295	Sales calls, marketing, general business
Administrative Assistant	1685	
Business Office	1884	Billing questions
Supervisor	1428	Problems/complaints
Letter A–G	1567	Billing question per last name
Letter H–P	1897	Billing question per last name
Letter Q–Z	1289	Billing question per last name
Transcription	1996	
Supervisor	1953	Referral letter
Physicians	1960	
Dr. Jones	1988	
Mary Jones, Medical Assistant	1991	Patient questions/problems
Dr. Youngblood	1435	
John Helper, Medical Assistant	1456	Patient questions/problems
Dr. Gilbert	1756	
Jenny Rebecca, Medical Assistant	1578	Patient questions/problems

TABLE 5-2

Telephone Call Transfer Log (Study)

Time Block	Dr. J	Dr. Y	Dr. G	Business Office	Administration
9 AM–10 AM	✓✓✓	✓✓✓	✓✓	✓	✓✓✓✓
10 AM–11 AM	✓	✓✓✓✓	✓✓	✓✓	✓✓✓✓
11 AM–12 PM	✓✓✓✓	✓✓	✓✓✓	✓✓✓✓	✓
12 PM–1 PM	✓✓	✓✓✓✓	✓✓✓	✓✓✓✓—✓✓✓✓	✓✓✓

From this log, a count report by hour and destination can be produced. From there, these data can be placed on a graph. The data have numerous uses, including:

- Staffing patterns for different departments. Heavy phone volumes (such as at the reception/operator location) may require additional staff.
- Work flow plans for departments. If calls are bunched at certain times of the day, staff must be assigned to make these incoming calls the priority over other activities.

The second key study to undertake is a "Busy Study." The local phone company usually will conduct this study, often at no charge. In this study, all calls coming into the practice are counted by discrete calls and time per call. The study uses phone company equipment to monitor the lines (not conversations!) and also can count those incoming calls that get a "busy" signal.

Most private phone systems can track call volumes by each line and in hour increments (if not smaller increments). There probably are peaks and valleys in your call volume and, by looking at these reports and drawing a graph, you can readily see these patterns. When your receptionist complains about the call volume, you now have the information to evaluate what you are being told.

Finally, many answering services have sophisticated telephone usage and message tracking systems. Ask your service to generate reports for you, and review them for times of calls, types of calls, types of complaints presented by the patients (i.e., reason for the call), and the disposition (reassured patient, prescribed drug, admitted to hospital, sent to ER, and so on). From these reports you can assess what assistance patients are looking for outside of the regular office hours.

From these three studies—telephone triage, call busy, and answering service usage—a practice now has the ability to analyze call patterns and assess the number of lines, the use of dedicated lines, and staffing patterns and work plans. A sample set of objectives of the completed telephone plan might include the following:

- All incoming calls will be answered by the third ring either by a person or the automatic attendant.

- Calls answered by automatic attendant will be answered by a human being within 20 seconds of the first answer.
- All calls that are transferred will be answered either by the destination person or a voice mail within three rings.
- Any call on hold for more than one minute at the destination location will "ring back" at the destination location; if not answered in three rings, the call will automatically transfer to the main reception point.
- All calls where a message is left will be answered within 24 hours. Patient calls will be answered within one hour. For the latter, this may represent a simple acknowledgment that the message has been received and the patient's concerns will be addressed.

Well, now the patient has managed to get through to the appointment person, who will schedule an appointment. Once the date and time is scheduled, the appointment person will need to ask the questions described on page 118.

With employment in turmoil, and health coverage in turmoil, it behooves you to always check the latest status of a patient's employer and health insurance. What you are looking for is an MCO plan that will require any previsit referral form, clearance, or other hoops to jump through. Let me make this simple: if you're a specialist, there are hoops. Start jumping! Knowing this, arm your staff with the ability to rapidly dial out—this means using speed dial for the commonly called plans and the redial feature (busy signals are common).

THE ACTUAL VISIT

After all this, there arrives the day when the patient comes to your office. The patient enters the office, confronting a small, windowless room with the frosted glass panels closed, and hears the muffled voices of the staff. After rapping on the glass or, more personally, signing a line on a clipboard, someone may or may not acknowledge that the patient is here and check him in. Patients should be acknowledged within 15 seconds of arrival, even if your staff needs to complete another task before helping them. This simple courtesy conveys the message that the patient is important. The visit provides a second opportunity to check the patient's address and employment. It is more effective to ask the patient his address, employment, and plan, because if you ask them, "Do you still work at WXY Corporation and live at 911 Hemostat Drive?" the patient may simply say "Yes," thinking, "I don't want to bother going through reregister." Again, this is the last checkpoint for specialists to make sure that a referral form is in hand. If there is no form, the bill may become "patient responsible." Some plans deem the patient to be responsible for obtaining and conveying the referral form, while other plans deem that the providers are the responsible party. As a practical matter, however, it falls upon the provider to make sure the form is present.

With multiple plans and multiple components of plans, depending upon the employer, the physician and the office staff need to have ready access to certain components of each plan. An MCO desk reference (Table 5–3) is an ideal method for providing key information in a readily readable format. Physicians have one set of needs, the medical assistants have another, and the front desk and appointment desk staff have other needs.

As you can see in Table 5–3, the front desk person can locate the carrier and the specific plan (which can be a general plan or a plan tailored to the employer), identify the copayment due at the time of service, and determine any specific plan requirements that need to be addressed at the front desk, such as a referral form.

The desk reference may be sorted by health plan, but it is very important to ask the patient's employer as well. Large employers are often self-insured, and the health plan acts as the third party administrator (TPA). The role of a TPA is to receive and process health claims, for which it is paid an administrative fee by the employer. When it comes time to pay claims, the TPA looks to the employer to transfer the funds. To the employees, it is a seamless transaction; often, they do not realize that their plan is self-insured.

This being said, there are of course numerous wrinkles. There can be literally dozens of plans out there all operating under the umbrella of one plan name. Practices have some means to protect themselves through preventative actions, the enforcement of clear policies, and ongoing communication with their patients.

TABLE 5–3

Front Desk Reference

Riverland MSO
Front Desk Reference
Employer/Carrier Key Information
As of: March 1, 1995

Employer	Carriers	Plan Type	Co-Pay	Other	Assignment?
IBM	IBM Employee H.P.	Indemnity	N/A	Prudential TPA	Y
	US Healthcare	HMO	$ 10		Y
	Aetna	PPO	$10/ $15		Y
State of NC	State Employee H.P.	Indemnity	N/A		N
	State Employee PPO	PPO	$7 /$20		N
United Teachers	NY Life	Indemnity	N/A		Y
	Healthsource	HMO	$ 5		Y
	US Healthcare	HMO	$ 15		Y
US Post Office	USPO Employ Health Plan	Indemnity	N/A		N
	BC Companion HMO	HMO	$0		Y

One of the best ways to address the financial issues is to give all patients a brochure outlining the financial policies of the practice. In the policy, you can outline some basic terms:

1. Billing for indemnity plans is a courtesy, unless the practice takes assignment.
2. Billing for HMOs and other managed care plans with whom you have a contract is for the services covered only. It is expected that the patient will understand what is covered and what is not.
3. All copayments will be collected at time of service.
4. Any coinsurance amounts will be billed after the plan has adjudicated the claim. Payment is then expected within 10 days.

If these policies, particularly the collection of copayments, represent a policy change for you (in other words, you had the sign on the desk but never enforced it), you will need to send nice letters to your patients telling them that, effective on such and such a date, you will always collect the copays at the time of service. Coupled with this policy, however, is the need to accept credit cards, if you haven't been doing so already. The acceptance of credit cards is so widespread in the United States (even grocery stores accept them) that this is generally a reasonable expectation. Accepting credit cards is a convenience to patients. You also will find that patients can use the card for paying coinsurance amounts, expensive test fees, and past due balances by phone.

Finally, you will need to begin to strictly enforce this policy. Enforcement includes beginning to turn patients away when they don't have the copayments with them. "We would be pleased to reschedule your appointment," you might say. During the transition period, it also would be helpful for the physicians to mention this to patients after the exam.

A note about copayments: it is expected that the copayment is due and payable at the time of service. Since the amount is small (typically $10 or $15), it would cost almost as much to bill this amount. Secondly, the MCO expects that the copayment will be paid at the time of service, and the member/patient must clearly understand that this is the expectation. You can fall back to that rationale, smilingly explaining to the patient that her health plan requires this copayment, and, yes, you do accept credit cards. Copayments can make up a significant amount of cash revenue, so do not let this slide.

Once past the "check-in," the patient is then asked to have a seat in the "reception room" (a different impression than "waiting room," isn't it?). Although the jokes are endless, try breaking the stereotype. Magazines can be ordered just for reception room use and can be discarded after two to three weeks. The selection of magazines can reflect the interests of your patients in addition to mindless material many people like while, well, waiting. A mix of "general interest," gender-oriented (e.g., *Woman's Day* versus *GQ*), local interest (e.g., city magazines such as *New York* or *Washingtonian*), and business (e.g., *Business Week* or *Forbes*) magazines is a good strategy. The local newspaper would be a nice touch. You also should mix in health newsletters, such as the Harvard letters, the Mayo Clinic Report, and brochures from your professional society, hospital, and special interest organizations (American Heart Association, American Cancer Society, and so on). Finally, with the rising need for elderly care and support from adult children, brochures and newsletters dealing with the subject of caring for parents, nursing home care, and Alzheimer's disease, to mention a few, also would be helpful. As an added service, you could offer to photocopy a specific article for patients (although be careful about running afoul of copyright laws).

There are many first impressions that a practice makes, and the reception room is just one. The most frightening reception room I ever saw occurred on a job interview. As I walked into the room, there, staring me in the face, were those posters—you know, the four or five employment posters about the minimum wage law, workers compensation, and the like that you're required to post for your employees. Most people put these a closet; here, they were on a reception room wall.

As a general rule, you would like your reception area to be comfortable. It should be well lit, although indirect lighting is easier for elderly patients. Carpets should not be overly busy; very busy patterns can be disorienting. Obviously, you should avoid pictures that might be regarded as sexist or otherwise in poor taste, including advertising calendars provided by drug companies. Importantly, leave areas open for wheelchairs to fit comfortably without blocking accesses; you can do what many movie theaters do, and simply remove seats. The chairs themselves should be functional, comfortable, and have arms. The arms are an aid to the elderly in general and to any patient who may need that "boost" to get up out of a chair.

And Now, the Moment We've Been Waiting For

The frosted glass door slides open, or the door pops open, and someone calls, "Rick?" Addressing patients, especially elderly ones, by their first names, unless you know them well or unless they have asked you to, is not considered good manners. The patient is now led back into the warren of rooms, and the actual visit begins. Often, the medical assistant will take the weight, temperature, and blood pressure, and ask how the patient is feeling. This is an important, but often underappreciated, encounter. Patients often will have a relationship with the office staff that is different than the one they have with the physician. The assistant spends more time with the patient, talks with him more frequently, and is privy to medical and sometimes financial details. The time the medical assistant spends with the patient, then, can be leveraged to bring the assistant into the treatment process by making her another pair of eyes and ears providing information and observations to the physician.

The assistants should have a standard set of tasks to perform for patients and specific questions to ask. Questions may include asking if patients are taking any other medication that another physician may have prescribed, how they are feeling in general, whether they have had the flu that's been going around, and so on. The assistant also can ask the patient about any questions or issues that they would like to discuss with the physician. Another way to help convey this information to the physician is to leave a clipboard in the reception room inviting patients to make a note of their questions and concerns. This can then serve as the basis of discussion with the physician during the visit.

This all said, if medical assistants are to be another set of eyes and ears to support the physician, they need to have a body of knowledge to do so. Medical assistants who have been through a training program will have some knowledge, but they will not necessarily possess the knowledge base specific to the specialty or focus of the practice. Continuing training, then, is a responsibility of the practice.

The objective of this training is simple: the more the staff understands what the physicians do, the more it can identify potentially significant comments made by patients, the more it can anticipate the physicians' needs in treating patients, and the more it can answer questions and interpret information that may be flowing through the medical assistants and to and from physicians, patients, and other physicians.

As an example, a training program for a practice might take the form of a "lunch and learn" arrangement—the practice can order sandwiches in for a lunch hour program. (Yes, you will have to pay the staff for this time.) Required attendees would include medical assistants, but all staff members (particularly transcriptionists) should also be invited. Topics might include:

- System anatomy related to the specialty.
- Common presenting problems and illnesses.
- Diagnostic tests (how the test is done, what is being looked for, what the different findings mean).
- Common medications used (their purpose and side effects).
- The physical exam (what is examined, what different findings mean, signs and symptoms).

A specialty practice may cover the material in fewer sessions than a general or primary care practice, because the scope of what may be presented to the physician is wider for the "generalist" practices.

Training is not a one-time event, however. One or two summary "update" sessions should be held on at least a quarterly basis. These sessions serve as a refresher for the staff, a time for the physicians to emphasize certain topics that are of most importance (or address seeming weaknesses on the part of the staff), as well as an opportunity to update the staff on new developments and advances that it should be aware of, such as new drugs or tests.

Hi! I'm Dr. Welby. How Are We Today?

We now return to the patient visit. After the initial vitals are taken by the medical assistant, the patient is then led into an examining room and told, "The doctor will be right with you." The patient is then left to wait. And wait. Managing a patient appointment schedule is difficult, at best, and always staying on time without shortchanging some patients is simply not possible. What is possible, however, is always being late. This is a simple enough concept—if the physician is always running late, then either the physician needs to change, or the schedule needs to change to accommodate his manner of practice. Practices that are always running behind schedule probably find that the patients start factoring in the tardiness and showing up late. Which puts you further behind. And so on, and so on.

When things are going wrong in serving your patient (and running late is one of the major offenses) the best defense is to come clean, take responsibility, and move on. If you're running behind, have the front desk staff tell the patients up front. If the physician has been legitimately called out of the office for an emergency, do have your staff try to reach patients and reschedule for either later in the day (which may involve extending office hours) or another day.

Some of the scheduling problems practices face result from plans promoted by consultants. Some of these schedule plans are so geared to the convenience of the office that they are a turnoff to patients. It is impossible to predict with certainty how long an individual patient will take—seemingly simple matters are actually complex, a new problem is presented at the last minute, or whatever. What irritates patients is not being told the truth. Being placed in an exam room, when you know full well that you will be waiting for some time, is cruel and unusual punishment, and patients are on to the game.

Some days just go badly. If there is a particularly bad day, your best remedy is to send out letters of apology with an explanation of what happened, such as that there was one patient who needed a lot of your attention. An apology letter would be a welcome surprise, if for no other reason than no one else does it. I once had a good occasion to send such letters. A practice I was working with had an imaging unit break down one day, causing the cancellation of several patients, some of whom had been injected with radioactive isotopes. The staff didn't think that letters were necessary, they told me, as members had already spoken to the patients and no one was complaining. I sent out letters to these patients anyway. In the letter, I apologized for having to cancel their exam, explained what had happened, that the practice was working closely with the manufacturer to make sure that the unit was repaired, and that, hopefully, there would be no further problems. The upshot? The letter was mentioned by two patients the next time that they came for a visit.

Another example of the power of an apology involved American Thermoplastics in Pittsburgh. I once had an occasion to order a $5 pocket calendar from the company. The order was placed in December, so I expected a delay, and my calendar was delivered in what I thought was fairly short order. Imagine my surprise, then, when I received a letter from the president of the company, apologizing for the delay in the shipment. Funny thing was, I didn't ever realize it was late!

My last example of an apology letter involves an airline. USAir had had an unfortunate string of five or so accidents, culminating in the fatal crash of a 737 on its final approach to Pittsburgh. Shortly afterward, a letter came from the chairman of the company to all frequent flyers. The letter hit the three key points:

- Express regret and remorse (if appropriate).
- State why the incident happened (if known).
- Explain what you're going to do to prevent a reoccurrence.

Here again, the impact of the letter was enhanced because of the simple fact that no one else does it! The USAir letter was direct, acknowledging the accidents, reporting that a retired U.S. Air Force general had been appointed to oversee safety throughout the company, and stating that if there was any doubt as to the safety of the fleet, the chairman would ground all of the planes.

When the physician is spending time face-to-face with a patient, the pressure is there to move quickly through the exam and discussion. The trick—a very difficult trick—is to move quickly while giving the impression that the patient has the physician's complete, undivided attention, and patient has all of the time she needs to discuss what's on her mind. As noted earlier in this chapter, one tool that a number of practices find effective is a form that prompts the patient to write out her questions or notes while in the reception area or before coming in to the office. You may find it effective to place such forms, already on a clipboard with a pen, at the front desk so that patients will be prompted to complete them as they check in (Figure 5–2). Other techniques include:

- When you ask a patient, "Do you have any questions?" use the technique professional speakers use. After you ask the question, wait, without speaking, and count to "10." People need time to formulate a question, and they are often reticent about asking the physician to repeat the instructions or admitting that they don't understand what was just "explained" to them.
- Use written instructions, particularly when more than one medication is involved or the sequencing is important.

In the course of the visit, the physician may want to implement a treatment plan that will require the use of a specialist or ancillary service. He will leave the exam room and ask "Mary" to please schedule Mr. Lawrence for a test, say, an MRI. For most patients, Mary would simply call Denber Hospital and schedule the exam. If the patient is covered by an HMO, however, it is critical for the practice and for the patient that the right referral be made. The usual providers with whom the practice does business may not be in the HMO's network.

So, Mary will need to pull out the MCO Fact Book, a binder that lies on the desk of every medical assistant. In this binder there is a page for each HMO and PPO that the practice contracts with, that clearly organizes the key information that the staff will need to be able to access quickly (Figure 5–3).

The physician has yet a different set of information needs. It is not material to him what the copayment is, nor does he need the details of making the referral.

FIGURE 5–2

Question Form

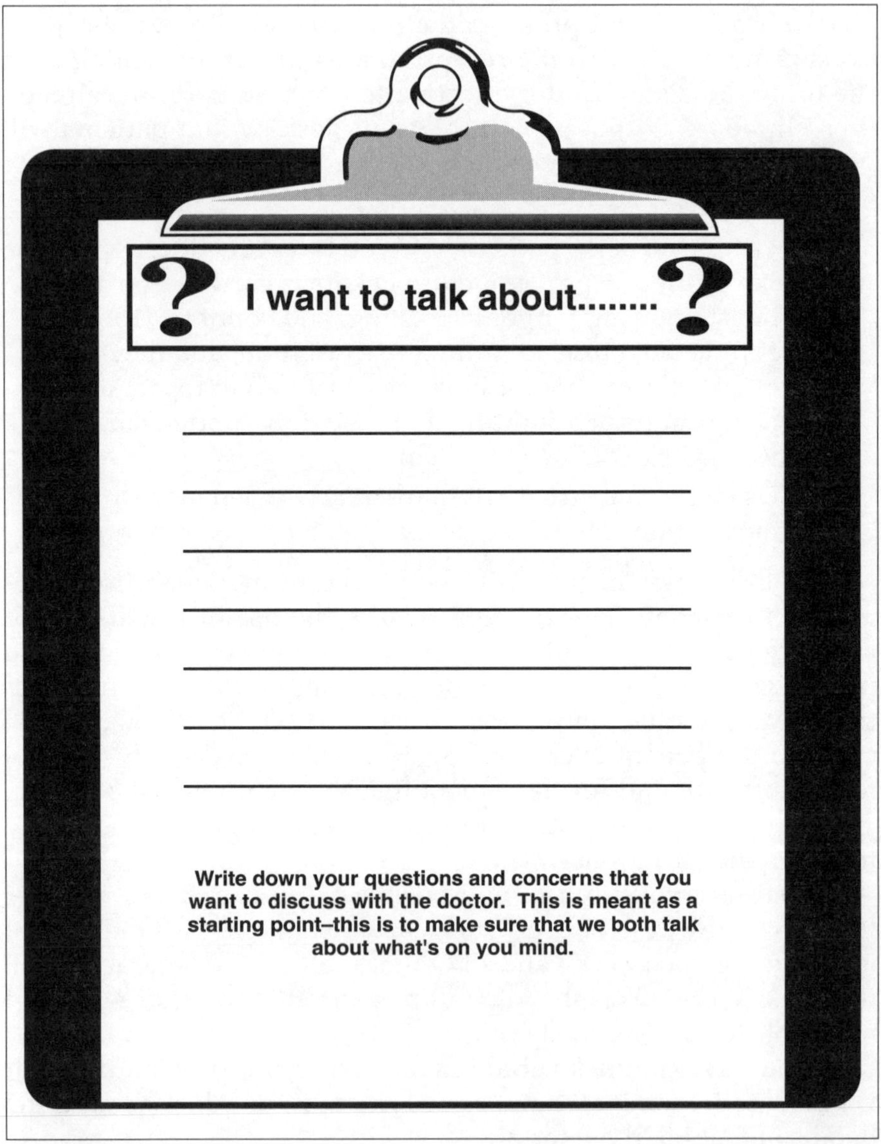

I want to talk about........

____

____

____

____

____

____

____

Write down your questions and concerns that you want to discuss with the doctor. This is meant as a starting point–this is to make sure that we both talk about what's on you mind.

FIGURE 5–3

MCO/Insurance Fact Reference Sheet

MCO/INSURANCE FACT REFERENCE SHEET

Billing Address:
10-20 Willie Sutton Boulevard
Truth or Consequences, NM
90796

PAY
$10/office visit

LAB and X-RAY
Lab: General Hospital
Appt.: call 833-9232
7:30AM – 4:00PM

X-ray: Routing in office OK
Specialist may order for inhouse or General Hospital outpatient

>>>> MRI: Get PCP referral

Advanced Diagnostic Radiology only
Appt.: Call 845-6000
7:30AM–7:00PM
Mon–Sat

OTHER TESTS
UR will advise when pre-authorization or pre-admit obtained

PLAN NAME:
Blinder Health Plan

UR Phone: 704-555-9334
Billing: 704-555-1212
Other: 704-555-1313

REFERRALS
PCP must approve and generate referral form
FAX copy acceptable

PRIOR AUTHORIZATION
Office procedures: Must be included in written referral form
OR
PCP verbal clearance OK
Document in chart

ALL INVASIVE PROCEDURES:
Contact PCP–PCP will obtain pre-authorization and make written referral

PRE-ADMISSION
Manadatory–PCP to arrange
Call UR 704-555-9334 if emergency admit only and PCP not reached

SECOND OPINION
See reverse of this Fact Sheet

It is important, however, for the physician to be aware of several contractual stipulations that impact his clinical decision making:

- Any restrictions on services that the practice would normally provide.
- Hospitals and imaging centers that must be used.
- Any limitations on prescription drugs.

Forms such as the physician MCO fact sheet (Figure 5–4) have been adopted by many practices on a formal as well as an ad hoc basis. The development of these forms is an ideal project to assign to the line staff, and you may find that there is already an informal system in use. Focusing on the organization and layout of the material and providing multiple copies so that the staff will have ready access to it will make these fact sheets a valuable resource.

CUSTOMER SERVICE

The notion of customer service in health care has been somewhat of an oxymoron. We talk about it, write articles and books about it, hire consultants, but just don't get it! We like to think our patients love us, that they have this bond—this very special, intimate relationship—we like to think that our patients will fight for us and fight to stay with us. We are shocked and very hurt when patients drop us because the big, bad managed care plan made them. Let me suggest that Marcus Welby is fiction. There are patients who do have that kind of relationship, but they are becoming more the exception. With so many physicians around, with demand dropping and supply increasing, patients can and will change physicians. One way to fight this and, more importantly, the managed care plans, is to deliver exceptional customer service. Impersonal attitudes from the staff mean impersonal care from the physicians.

As physicians are coming to be held accountable and responsible for what they do, they also are being held to a higher standard as to *how* they do what they do. This is the customer service aspect of medical care. With patient satisfaction such an important factor in measuring quality of care, the entire "flower" of services

FIGURE 5-4

Physician MCO Fact Sheet

Riverland Cardiology Group
MCO/Insurance Desk Reference
As of Sept. 1, 1994

PHYSICIAN
DESK
REFERENCE

PLAN (UR Tel. #)	Referral Form	Spec. Refer?	Ancillary Svcs In-House	Lab	X-Ray	Prior Author	Pre Admiss. Approval	Form-ulary	Hospital
Chuck's	Y	Y	Y	Gen Hosp	Advanced	Y	Y	N	Gen Hosp
800.322.5393				Radiology					Kaye Gen
Bill's	Y	N	N	Morgantown	Gen Hosp	Y	Y	N	Gen Hosp
202.444.1212`				Pathology	MRI Call UR				
Blinder Hlth Pl	N	N	N	Brennen	Robinson	Y	Y	N	Sancho
914.555.1111				Labs	Radiology				Memorial

Staff Desk Reference will include copay requirements, telephone numbers of membership verification desk, and other pertinent information

Fact Sheet contains more detailed information.

FIGURE 5–5

Flower of Service

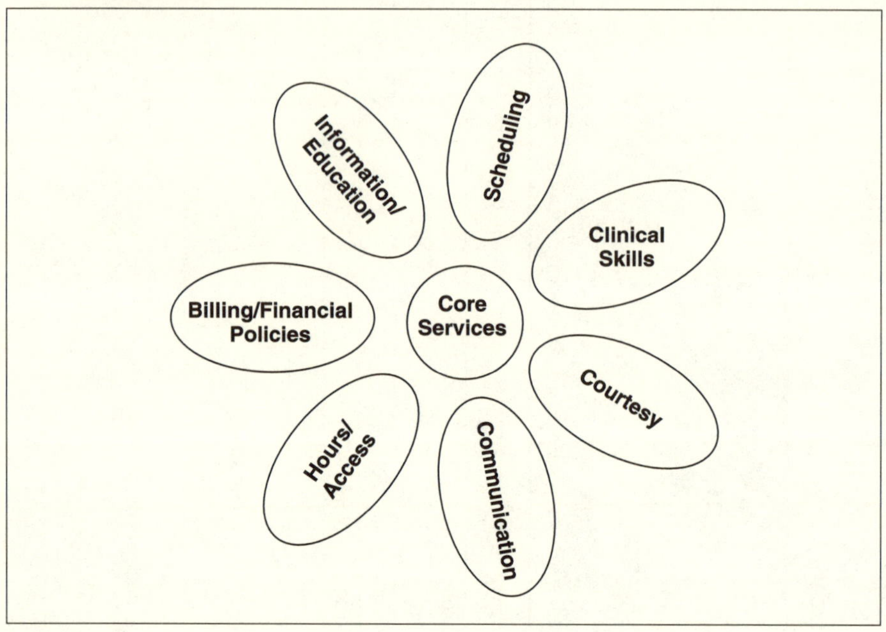

Adapted from ideas of C. Lovelock, "Planning Review" Jul/Aug 1995

that impacts a patient's visit has an impact on the quality of care. I define customer service in the broadest terms of the relationship between the physician, the practice operations, and the patient. It is this entire experience, or set of experiences, that drives patient satisfaction and the quality of care (Figure 5–5).

Customer service for the practice encompasses every interaction between the practice, the patient, the patient's family, and yes, the patient's insurer. It begins from the first point of contact, usually the phone, and continues through every interaction through the patient's discharge from the practice whether through end of illness, relocation, patient choice, or death. Consider for a moment the number of interactions that occur in a simple office visit, as presented in the chart below. This chart is basic in its description. In a simple office visit, the patient can interact with five or more people; use the phone system, the computer system, and its various modules (billing, appointment); rely on a medical records clerk to have the proper forms and reports filed in the proper medical records so they are in place in the exam room when the physician meets the patient; and so on. There are easily 25 or more interactions that can take place in the course of a visit. Here, I've only looked at the five specific actions that encompass a simple visit (Table 5–4).

Start counting the number of interactions in Table 5–4—*and I've simplified all this!* All of these interactions, taken together, are how patients view the care they receive from the practice. Computer systems that don't respond, medical records that either aren't available or aren't up-to-date, and billing statements that are in "code" all contribute to a frustration and lack of satisfaction.

Looked at in its entirety, the time spent with the physician is only a small part of the total time of a patient's visit. There is probably more time spent waiting than there is time spent doing anything else. From a patient's perspective, her interaction with the practice is through the office staff, whose members serve as eyes, ears, translators, and advisors for the patient. Few physicians answer their own phones; in most instances, a patient has to get through the office staff in order to get to the physician. Patients also know that in order for their concerns to be given priority, they must stay on the good side of the staff. The staff can either go out of its way for the patient or take the bureaucratic stonewall approach and stall or delay action.

The physician sets the tone for the practice or its culture, if you will. The level of importance placed on messages, proper phone answering, message taking, and such all set the tone of the practice and are part of the customer service aspect. This happens in many ways, many of which may be unconscious. Consider, for example, how the physician reacts to a stack of phone messages from patients, whether he scowls and grumbles at the calls to make or views them as one of the ways that he cares for patients. A physician who makes derogatory comments about Medicaid or Medicare patients is sending a clear message to his staff that he considers them to be second class people, not deserving of respect or consideration. Worse, the physician who groans when the phones are ringing, or when he has to talk to a family member about a hospitalized patient, is one who sends the message that patients are an annoyance.

TABLE 5-4

Patient/Staff Interactions During an Office Visit

Event	Staff Interaction	System Interaction	Actions
Appointment call	Telephone operator Scheduler/ appointment clerk	Phone system Computer system	Call answered, transferred On hold tape System responds appointment available and convenient Entered correctly
Visit/ reception	Receptionist	Computer System	Patient acknowledged immediately Greeted within 15 seconds System responds Appointment correct
		Waiting room	Waiting room clean Current magazines, materials
	Medical records technician	Medical records	Record up-to-date, available for staff
Exam		Facility layout, ambiance, temperature control	No long walks Handicap access Clean Comfortable environment
	Medical assistant		Greets patient Preliminary history, vitals
		Exam room equipment	Exam room clean, ready
	Physician		Greets patient Conducts appropriate exam Answers/anticipate questions Writes instructions—gives to medical assistant
Checkout	Business office clerk	Computer system Billing software/forms	Patient greeted and checked out promptly
	Appointment clerk	Computer system Forms Recall system Reminder system	System responds, current data Prints readable form New appointment made Enter data for reminder
Follow-up	Physician	Mail Medical records	Physician reviews results within 24 hours of arrival
	Medical assistant	Phone/mail	Test results are communicated to patient within 24 hours of arrival
		Medical records	Results posted to medical record

I'll say it: "Make the patient the focus of the practice." Physicians face real competition in their practices today, facing fewer patients and declining income. As with any business, the way to compete is to focus on what you're doing—and what practices do is care for patients. Creating a practice that is patient focused is not simply a matter of spouting pithy phrases. It's about culture, behavior, attitudes, business processes and policies, and procedures.

I've never seen a practice that wasn't overworked, understaffed, and had too many interruptions. People can puff themselves up and try to appear to be so important by being "too busy." Being too busy for your patients will be the death knell of your practice. The ones that break the mold, that focus on the patient, are the ones that, in the end, will thrive and succeed. Given a choice, people will rebel against indifference or arrogance.

A final thought about complaints: take them very seriously. Someone has commented that it is the patients (customers) who complain who are your best patients, because they care enough to say something. In the marketing chapter (Chapter 9), we will discuss patient satisfaction studies, a valuable tool for assessing the state of the relations with your patients.

In Chapter 9 we will also discuss a number of techniques of creating a practice that looks and acts with the focus on the patient. Marketing, as will be discussed, is not advertising, but is composed of four components: product, price, place, and promotion (which includes, but is not exclusively, advertising). These are known as the "four Ps" of marketing.

BILLING AND CLAIMS FILING

Billing a managed care plan in many ways is no different than billing any other indemnity carrier. Preventative care and "Don't play the victim" are the two bywords which can be suggested. Unlike your relationship with an indemnity plan, your relationship with a managed care plan is defined by the formal contract that you will have negotiated and signed. With this contract, then, there is a relationship, one that sets a different level of participation and communication than has historically been the case. Many practices have difficulty getting used to the idea that they have a different relationship, that when they bill the MCO, they are filing the practice's claim, not doing the patient a favor by filing the claim.

As you recall, part of the purpose of the due diligence is to prepare for implementing the contract. When a contract is being signed and implemented, your billing staff or lead billing person should arrange to meet with the claims staff at the managed care organization in order to ensure that claims processing will be handled properly. If the MCO handles claims processing at a distant site, a telephone conference call can be arranged in many instances. In proposing and setting up the meetings, you are conveying to the MCO staff that:

- You are used to managed care.
- You want to make sure that claims are processed properly.
- You simply want to go through a checklist and review procedures to make sure you are following the procedures required by the MCO.

Your attitude and presentation should be one of being helpful, open, cooperative, and very supportive of the mutual goals of the MCO and yourself. As with many things in life, it is always helpful if you have a personal relationship with your counterpart. In the due diligence stage discussed earlier, I suggested that you in fact have the name of a key contact person at the MCO in the event of billing problems. Under capitation you may still be required to file claims with the insurance carrier.

Importantly, under HMOs you may find that your preventative care visits are now reimbursable. Historically, under the standard indemnity plans, preventative care services such as immunizations, screening, and the general annual checkup were not reimbursed. Well-baby visits are an example. Under HMOs there tends to be an emphasis on preventative care, which was the underlying rationale behind HMOs in their early days. Whether a negotiated fee-for-service or a capitation situation in which claims are still being filed, do inquire with your carrier whether by billing and using preventative medicine codes you will be paid or credited for rendering a covered service. As has been noted, many HMOs not only pay for but actively encourage immunizations and screenings. They may even use the percentage of your patients who have received their immunizations and screenings on time as one tool of measuring quality care and, in some instances, pay bonuses for achieving certain targets. As an example, 85 percent of the children in a certain age bracket may have received their immunizations on time.

The ICD-9 diagnosis codes, which stand for the international classification of diseases, are also updated yearly. It is important to code to the fifth digit where possible, as more carriers are looking for a definitive diagnosis. Be aware also, particularly with Medicare, that for certain procedures and testing, they will be looking for certain diagnosis codes in order to justify the service being rendered, so it is important that complete and accurate coding be done.

You still may be required to file a claim, even under capitation, for various reasons, among them utilization tracking, budget caps, and the like. Plans are looking for over-utilization, inappropriate services being rendered, and unnecessary services being rendered, even in situations where there is a capitation contract. The plans ultimately are looking to ratchet down utilization in the plans. Be aware that, as utilization comes down, they may approach you and suggest a lower capitation rate, since you are providing fewer services than initially projected.

6 CHAPTER

Financial Management

The saying is that there are three important things in real estate: location, location, location. In running any small business such as a practice, there also are three important things: cash, cash, cash. Professional practices such as a medical practices are labor intensive and generally supported by little capital investment relative to the size of the organization. The greatest asset they have are the people who work there: physicians, technical staff, and all support staff. The adage, "Your assets walk out the door every night," is quite apt here. Additionally, as a professional practice, the financial capital necessary to operate and invest in the practice and its future can only come from working capital generated within the practice or debt. Nonphysicians cannot invest and own stock in a professional practice. The practice management companies discussed earlier do have the means to get around this requirement, but that opens up another series of decisions for the practice to undertake. For the purpose of our discussion here, we will focus on the self-sustaining practice.

Managed care does require more overhead and intensive management to manage successfully. At the same time, fees and revenue are coming down, putting a squeeze on a declining profit margin. When practices experienced profit margins of 40 to 50 percent, the margin of error was such that swings in practice revenue would have minimal impact on the survivability of a practice. But as profit margins have become smaller and smaller, the margin of error also has become smaller and can put a practice at more serious risk of running into serious financial trouble. Such swings in revenue and profitability can throw a practice into a loss situation.

Successful financial management of a practice comes down to a few key rules:

- Bill promptly, electronically, and often.
- Never be a victim—fight the good fight!
- Follow the money trail.
- Watch the pennies.
- Invest in your practice.

The flip side of a successful practice in a managed care world is the ability to apply business skills to the running of the practice. As with any organization, financial management is one of the two or three critical components, along with the product and marketing and the management team. Financial management encompasses a wide range of activities, all of which deal with the conservation and utilization of the assets of the practice. In this chapter, I will lay out a number of tools with which to accomplish this responsibility.

The keeping of the financial records of the practice has two purposes: (1) to provide information for management decision making; and (2) to determine tax and other regulatory obligations. As you develop plans to implement some of the techniques outlined here, do make sure that you consult with your accountant wisely to make sure that what you do to provide or enhance management information does not interfere with or otherwise complicate the compilation of records and reports for taxes, lenders, or other needs.

In assessing your practice's financial management, one of the first steps is to assess your accountant: does this person possess the technical accounting knowledge, an understanding of how medical practices operate, and the business experience to advise you on the range of financial and management issues that arise in your practice? You are looking for someone with more than technical knowledge; you are looking for someone who can apply the technical knowledge in a business setting, to real situations, constraints, and trade-offs. In your assessment of and search for an accountant, it is entirely appropriate to meet and interview potential advisors, in much the same way you would interview a potential employee.

The third, and possibly most important, aspect to look for in an accountant is how comfortable you feel with the person, and how much you trust her judgment. This is as much personality as experience and know-how. This is a highly personal relationship—what works for one person may not work for another.

A very big caution: physicians, for whatever reason, sometimes end up with "advisors" who would be better off left at a carnival sideshow. We've all heard the stories, some more horrifying than others. I've seen contracts that should never have been signed—that attorneys have advised their clients to sign. Physicians are magnets for every investment and "get rich quick" scheme, in that many outsiders are under the impression that all physicians have nothing but money and are always willing to invest. Many, if not most, physicians are well aware of this and are on guard but, still, scam artists and bad advisors slip through the cracks. For reasons such as this, the time you spend finding the right set of advisors will be of enormous value to you in the future.

MANAGING YOUR CASH

As noted above, the most important aspect of financial management is the management of cash. As with any business, you can be profitable on the books, but if the cash isn't there to make payroll, purchase raw materials, and pay vendors, you're out of business.

The management of cash begins at the time of the patient visit. Medical practices carry very heavy accounts receivable loads, due to the common practice of having to bill insurance carriers and wait for payment. Because of this, the monies that you should be collecting at the time of service *really need to be collected at the time of service!* As has been discussed in earlier chapters, it is critical for the practice to collect insurance information and copayments up front at the time of service. Since the name of the game is cash, the sooner you collect it, the better off you are.

One of the ways to enhance your cash collection is to accept credit cards. Credit card payments are "good" funds in your bank account within 48 hours after the ticket is submitted to the bank for clearing. In addition to aiding the collection of copayments at the time of service, credit card payments can be taken by mail or phone. Once the EOB has been returned from the carrier with the patient's responsibility (coinsurance, copayment, deductible, whatever), a phone call can generate the collection simply by the patient authorizing a charge to his credit card. If done by mail, patients can simply settle their account with you immediately. To accomplish this, enclose a special charge form with your statement, or preprint the credit card information form on the back of the return portion of your statement, including a signature line. A practice also can have the patient authorize an immediate charge to her card when the EOB is issued for any charges still due. The authorization can include a dollar cap as well. You may surprised as to the volume of charges that are settled by credit card. I was.

As an aside, Visa has a unit set up that specializes in serving medical practice accounts. The unit offers collection tips, forms, a video, and other items at no or low cost.

To accept charge cards, you will need to establish a "merchant account" with a bank. Most commercial and many savings banks can do this for you. The fees for setting up an account are nominal, but do shop around. There will be nominal charges to rent the embosser and electronic swipe to obtain authorizations, and you will need a phone line for handling the modem and authorizations. The major charge is the "discount rate," which typically will be between 1 and 4 percent for Visa and Mastercard, and up to 7 percent for American Express. The discount rate is the fee (determined as a percentage of each charge) that the bank charges in return for clearing the credit card charges. The discount rate is negotiable; it is based upon the average number of charge tickets per month and the average dollar value per ticket. Since your volume will undoubtedly increase as patients get used to using the card, make sure you go back and renegotiate the rate. Most practices will stick with Visa and MasterCard, which are the ones most commonly carried. American Express generally carries a higher "discount rate." American Express and the Discover Card may be worth consulting to see what kind of offer they will make; it may be beneficial to accept those cards if the demand is there from your patients.

Once the patient has been served, an accounts receivable has been created that will stay on the books until payments have been made. The practice's internal paper handling process must insure that all superbills/encounter forms are bundled and sent directly to the business office at the close of the day. It then falls upon the business office to make sure that the bill goes out promptly to the carrier. I have seen practices that take as long as a month before a claim is submitted. Claims need to be processed, ready to go, and out the door within 24 hours of the date of service. While some practices, because of low volume, may not bill more than once or twice a week, practices with a higher volume may be billing as much as once every day or repeatedly during the day, particularly if electronic billing is available.

It is an ongoing task to watch your financial and cash status on every day. I'm a fanatic for advocating daily cash monitoring for most businesses, and the advent of telephone bank reporting and now on-line information access make this an easy task. Using my own case as an example, on a daily basis, my assistant would call the bank's automated telephone system and check on the book balance, the available funds, and the funds that would become available on each of the next three business days. By obtaining this data, I could plan the practice's cash availability against its cash needs and budget accordingly. Depending upon your bank, these different levels of information are available. As computer banking comes on line, it will be possible to obtain more and more information using a computer with a modem.

By projecting forward several days, I could insure that cash would be available for payroll, for which available funds must be present in order to cover paychecks to be issued. When you use direct deposit, funds must be available on the pay date, since "clearing" is instantaneous. Secondly, it can take two to three days for even a small practice to prepare, record, and mail the accounts payable. I like to review the accounts payable on Wednesday, and, using the cash flow information, set a budget for payables. From there, I select those bills for payment that week or for that run. Checks are prepared and signed on Thursday and then checked again, and mailed on Friday. Before the final release of checks, I insure that all checks can be covered by available funds on the Monday when many will be arriving at the vendors' addresses and entering the banking system.

To keep track of all this, I used the form that follows (Figure 6–1). It is but one type of cash reporting form that I used on a weekly basis.

The cash availability in a given week also would account for the total accounts payable. Just because a bill is presented does not mean it is going to be paid immediately. In addition, reserves would be set aside for the quarterly or annual malpractice insurance payments and other predictable large expenses. Depending upon cash position and the payment terms, a budget was set for payables and the invoices to be paid that week were selected. If it was a payroll week, funds were reserved for the estimated payroll. What was left was what I prefer to call ADI, or available for distribution and investment. I refer to this as ADI rather than profit because the fact that it is leftover cash at a given point in time does not mean it is available to be distributed to the partners or otherwise used. These funds may need to have reserves set on them. Some organizations like to set up a separate bank account to hold funds in reserve for installment payments. If sufficient amounts of cash are available, you can move monies to money market funds, which may pay a slightly higher rate of interest. This often can be done electronically, which is where the only benefit truly comes in, since you have immediate access to your cash if you need it. With much larger sums and larger practices, banks have the ability to "sweep" an account daily, meaning that cash is put into overnight or very short-term (one-, two-, or three-day commercial paper) investments and moved back into the checking account to cover the checks being presented for payment on a given day. There are fees involved with all of this, and your bank can tell you what you have the ability to do.

Another technique to improve your cash flow if you have sufficient mail is to use a post office box and get the mail in the morning. Mail delivered to a post office box is typically available by 8:30 AM, which gives your staff all day to open the mail, record the checks, and get a deposit in the bank before the banking day cutoff. Many banks end their day as early as 2:00 PM, so any deposits

FIGURE 6–1

Cash Plan/Budget Form

Cash Position Statement and Plan for Week Ending ____________

Cash:

Check account balance:	____________
Available funds:	____________
Other cash funds:	____________

Total Cash Available:

Cash Commitments:

Accounts payable:	____________
Payables budget:	____________
Payroll:	____________
Partner distribution:	____________
Other:	
____________	____________

Total Cash Commitments:

ADI (Available for distribution and investment):

Billed:	____________	**Rate of:**	____________
Collected:	____________	**Rate of:**	____________

Approved: ________________________

Administrator

made, say, on a Monday after 2:00 PM are credited in the bank for Tuesday. There is then the float, which depends on how many days the bank must hold the funds, which in turn depends upon which part of the country the check comes from. This can amount to an additional three days. For example, a check deposited Monday at 3:00 PM would be considered by this bank as being deposited on Tuesday. Add three more days: Wednesday, Thursday, Friday. It is not until the following Monday, a week after receipt, that the check then becomes good funds. I encountered this situation with Medicare checks, which, although physically printed and processed in the state of New York, were drawn off a bank in Indianapolis, Indiana, which resulted in a three-day hold. As a consequence, it was often as much as a week before I would have the available funds. Depositing all checks and cash on the day received (as both a security issue as well as a cash flow issue) and accepting credit cards will improve your cash flow.

The management of the finances of a practice focuses on cash and assets to maximize their value and productivity. Finances are very much central to management activity. A stable financial base can lead to a smoothly running organization but, conversely, an unstable financial base can lead to dissension, discomfort, and turmoil. As Samuel Johnson once said, "If you ain't got the money, you gotta think." Next, we will deal with some of the central management tasks in the finance function of a practice.

DEVELOPING A BUDGET

While many managers are taught to focus on planning issues, one of the financial planning issues we are familiar with is the budget. Small practices typically will not have any sort of budget process, nor for that matter any kind of formal financial reporting process. Fundamentally, a budget is a detailed plan expressed in quantitative terms that specifies how resources will be acquired and used in a specified period of time, typically one year. A budget is a plan that forecasts the revenues and expenses of the organization. It is a means of allocating the organization's resources. That is, the projected cash revenue can be distributed to the owners as profit, used to make pay raises, invested in new capital equipment or a new piece of diagnostic equipment, used to expand facilities, or invested in capital equipment, such as computers and desks, to enable a practice to function and operate more efficiently and smoothly. A budget provides a means of control over the operations of the organization. It is also a means of measuring and evaluating its performance on a financial basis.

There are two basic types of budgets: an operating budget and a capital budget. An operating budget is a plan for the day-to-day operations of the organization, such as payroll, insurance expenses, telephone expenses, utilities, office supplies, and the like. A capital budget is a plan for the acquisition and disposal of capital assets. Capital assets typically have a life of over three years and cost more than $500. Typical capital assets include land, buildings, and certain equipment. However, don't confuse this discussion of the capital budget with the definitions used for tax purposes. For tax purposes, you may be able to expense an item that is technically a capital item. An EKG machine, for example, which has a long life, is a capital expense. Yet smaller practices may be able to treat the purchase cost as an expense for tax purposes.

In developing a budget, you are developing a projection of what will happen 12 to 18 months in the future. Obviously, a budget is not going to be 100 percent on the mark, unless you get very, very lucky. So in order to develop a good budget you need to make certain assumptions regarding estimated revenues, expenses, and business conditions; it is the soundness of these underlying assumptions that will determine the accuracy of the budget you develop. It should be noted here that budgets are not developed in stone, that they are subject to change and revision during the course of the year. In later pages we will discuss some of the pros and cons of how to handle this, but I am putting to rest the notion that, "If it is not in the budget, it can't be done." If it is not in the budget but you need to make an investment or incur an expense anyway, the budget is your basis for understanding the implication of your decision.

Among the assumptions necessary to develop a budget for a professional practice are the units of service. These can be estimated by procedure code but this may be fairly impractical. The more refined and precise the level of detail you are trying to predict and project, the more likely that you will make more significant errors. It makes more sense and is a sound business practice to do your projections by lines of service, such as office visits (which may be divided by new patients and current patients), lab, X-ray, hospital visits, emergency room visits, certain testing, and so on. The principle here is that there be some sort of rational division, which probably will be predicated by how you think about visits and services now. You also may look at different payers since this also will have an impact on your revenue. Managed care plans obviously will be paying fewer dollars than will standard indemnity plans or self-pay patients. You may apply a simple formula that assumes that 20 percent of your patients are, for example, HMO members. Therefore, you will assume that 20 percent of your services are for HMO members and reduce your revenue from your regular collections to the percentage that the HMOs end up paying.

A word of caution about trending (the use of the historical change in utilization as a predictor of the future). Accounting information and historical data are very important because they show you how services have been growing or declining over time. Based on that information, you can develop a trend line to see the differences from year to year or from six-month or quarterly periods. Regardless, you cannot assume that any particular trend is going to continue. This is where your assumption about business conditions comes in, that is, your assumption that you are going to see increases in some areas, decreases in other areas, or a flattening in yet other areas. I have even gone so far as to make projections by line of service and then reduce my collections by 10 percent because I just did not think, because of the way the numbers flowed out, that was in fact what would happen to the practice. To my astonishment and delight, this turned out to be a correct assumption. Keep in mind that it is better to be on the conservative side and project slightly low than it is to project slightly high or dramatically high on what you think might happen. Since we are in such turmoil in our industry, my recommendation is that you proceed on a conservative basis.

The second area where assumptions need to be made regards expenses. Your expense budget can be produced to a large degree using historic data, because expenses tend not to swing wildly from year to year unless a management decision has been made that will have an impact on expenses. If you are planning to upgrade your computer equipment, a management decision has been made, and you can plug in the cost of this upgrading into your expenses. It should not be a surprise; unlike your revenue, it is a predictable and controllable event. I recommend that you create four schedules as you build your assumptions for the expense budget.

The first is the *position control register.* Rather than a listing of employees, the best way to manage your practice is to start with a listing of its job positions. An individual employee is slotted into one of the job positions in the organization. From a management and budget perspective, this position exists regardless of whether an employee is actually filling it at this time or the position is vacant. This document, then, is a roster that lists every job by job position, as illustrated in Table 6–1. While in a small practice you are more concerned with the individual, what you really need to look at from a management perspective is the number of job positions that you are allowing in order to staff your practice. The person actually occupying that position is less relevant. For budgeting purposes, you need to budget the dollars to pay a person who will be occupying that job, regardless of who that person is. If a position is vacant at the time the budget year will begin, you will still want to budget dollars for that position because once you fill it you will be paying somebody. If you are planning to add additional staff, you would add the positions to the roster, note them as vacant, and calculate the dollars you will be paying the employees who will fill those positions, adjusting the dollars for the estimated time period when the positions will be filled. (As an example, for a calendar year budget, a new position that will not be filled until June will only be budgeted for half the projected annual salary.) Be careful, however, about midyear hires or new positions that will not require a full year's salary. In subsequent years, these positions will consume full year wages, and they can result in a significant increase in your expenses without a corresponding increase in revenue to support both the expense and the desired profit.

Above all, do not forget to account for overtime. Some positions have "scheduled" overtime that is routine and predictable. My preference, however, is to budget for overtime on a gross basis because you cannot always determine in advance who and what job position will be accruing overtime in the course of the year. I like to set a percentage of budgeted wages or a dollar number as my overtime budget. During the year, the payroll register records wages paid and overtime separately, so that I can track overall overtime wages against the overall budget. Again, remember, the position control register is designed to drive the budget, the financial reports, and the cash planning for the organization.

As can be seen in Table 6–1, each job is assigned a number. As a practice gets bigger, it may assign a prefix number that designates the department or the class of positions, such as all medical assistants start with "200", all receptionists with "100", and so on. The "standard hours" of the number of hours normally scheduled in a pay period. Any hours above the standard would be counted in the "overtime" line in the budget, even if the person is still on straight time. The purpose of the "overtime" line is to account for additional hours above standard. When budgeting the dollars, make sure that sufficient dollars are accounted for at the rate of time and a half. The "date authorized" column notes when the position was created by the practice. No person can be hired unless there is an open position.

Finally, do not forget to account and budget for the employer portion of payroll taxes, which includes Social Security taxes (at 7.652 percent currently) and state and federal employment taxes, such as unemployment insurance and short-term disability. The employee portion of these taxes is included in each employee's wages. The monies you withhold are the employee's monies, not your's. The practice, as the employer, acts as a collecting agent by withholding the monies and depositing them together with the employer's portion with the Internal Revenue Service (IRS). At all costs, make sure that these deposits are made and made on time. Since the employer is acting as an agent for the employee in withholding the taxes with the responsibility of transferring the monies to the IRS, if an employer fails to make the deposit, it is effectively stealing the money.

Having dealt with the IRS on behalf of a client who missed tax deposits, let me assure you that the IRS is not pleasant about such an action. The penalties for failure to make the deposit on time are stiff, and those penalties accrue (in addition to interest) rapidly and geometrically—and for good reason, as noted above.

A second schedule to prepare is a *schedule of insurance.* In this schedule, all insurance coverage is to be listed (Table 6–2).

TABLE 6–1

Position Control Register

Riverland Cardiology Associates
Position Control Register
30-Sep-96

Job No.	Title	Status: Filled (Name) Vacant	Stand. Hours	Pay Rate	Date Auth.	Annual Pay
100-01	Receptionist	Beverly, B.	80.0	$6.40	1/1/92	$13,312
100-02	Receptionist	Adams, R.	40.0	$6.40	1/1/92	$6,656
200-01	Med Assist	Jones, B.	80.0	$9.00	1/1/92	$18,720
200-02	Med Assist	Vacant	80.0	$10.00	1/1/92	$20,800
200-03	Med Assist	Bryan, T.	20.0	$7.50	1/1/92	$3,900
200-04	Med Assist	Pollard, T.	60.0	$8.30	1/1/92	$12,948
300-01	Business Off	Ireland, K.	80.0	$8.75	1/1/92	$18,200
300-01	Business Off	Parker, S. J.	80.0	$8.50	1/1/92	$17,680
400-01	Lab Tech	Chambers, D.	40.0	$12.00	1/1/92	$12,480
400-01	Nuclear Tech	Sesta, M.	60.0	$31.50	1/1/92	$49,140
500-01	Administrator	Green, A.	80.0	$26.33	1/1/92	$54,766
600-01	Physician	Tarnower, H.	80.0	$37.50	1/1/92	$78,000
600-02	Physician	Fleishman, J.	80.0	$37.50	1/1/92	$78,000
600-03	Physician	Suzanne, A.	80.0	$37.50	1/1/92	$78,000
Total			**940.0 Hrs/Period**	**$247.18 Per Period**		**$462,602 Per Annum**

TABLE 6–2

Schedule of Insurance

Policy Type	Value/ Limits	Carrier	Agent/ Broker	Premium	Renewal Date
Worker's comp					
Property					
General liability					
Professional liability					
Employee health					
Others (specify)					
Total					

For each policy, call the agent and inquire as to the range of increases that are being instituted by the carriers for policies such as your's. Pay particular attention to employee benefit policies, such as health insurance, which are prone to significant increases and can represent large dollar amounts.

The next schedule to prepare is a *schedule of leases.* This schedule includes all leases that are the responsibility of the practice, including any equipment leases for computers, diagnostic testing equipment, and the like, as well as for the rent on facilities. The sample format (Table 6–3) shows the information to be included, such as: date of origin, monthly payment, ending date, and buyout amount (should you choose to purchase the equipment at the end of the lease).

Remember also that, eventually, leases do run out. You must monitor the timing of leases so that you can make arrangements for when a lease expires. Your options include:

- Purchase the equipment for the "buyout amount" that has been established in the lease agreement.
- Extend the lease, although at a lower monthly payment (since the item has been depreciated and essentially paid out).
- Return the leased item and replace it with a new item and a new lease.

TABLE 6–3

Schedule of Leases

Type	Payment/ Month	Lease Origin Date	End Date	Renew or Return
Facility				
Computers				
Treadmill				
X-ray				
	(Total/Month)			

The cost-of-maintenance agreements for leased equipment are not a lease item in themselves because they will by and large continue regardless of whether you are still leasing the equipment or not. Maintenance and other repair and maintenance costs—routine, ongoing expenses—are treated as expenses as opposed to being capitalized. The value or outcome of the repair and maintenance service is of limited concern, as all equipment needs to be maintained in order to operate properly. These costs, then, should be listed as separate line items in the budget. As you are preparing your budget, call the leasing companies or maintenance companies (if under a maintenance contract) for an indication of what the pricing will be like in the course of the year for your budget purposes.

The last schedule is for *capital equipment* purchases being planned. If you are going to be paying cash for capital equipment, you need to make sure the cash is available. If you are going to be leasing, you will need to account for the estimated lease costs in your budget.

A schedule of capital equipment as shown in Table 6–4, is also a planning tool, presenting a means of systematically compiling a list of capital equipment to plan for replacement either in the coming year or the future. It can also be used to develop a "wish list" and selecting which projects to go ahead with and which to set aside. Acquiring capital equipment is an investment decision for the practice—remember the "I" in ADI? These costs, which can be significant, have an impact on the revenue and expense plan for the practice.

TABLE 6-4

Schedule of Capital Equipment

Name/ Description	Date Placed in Service	Purchase Price	Lease/Loan Payment	Payoff Date	Estimated Life	Replacement Cost
Existing						
EKG	6/22/91	$4,000		7/94	6 yrs	$7,000
Treadmill	8/22/87	$16,000		7/92	10 yrs	$20,000
Computer #92-1	6/92	$3,500		7/95	7 yrs	$2,200
Computer #92-2	6/92	$3,500		7/95	7 yrs	$2,200
Total		**$27,000**				**$31,400**

With these four schedules in place, you can then move on to developing the revenue and expense budget.

To develop a revenue forecast, start by looking at your past utilization by common procedure terminology (CPT) code. Your objective is to focus on the quantity of services rendered, not the specific CPT code fees. From the historic data, you can look for trends in your practice and develop projections for the coming year. Are you growing or decreasing? Where are your patients coming from? In developing your projections, some of the factors to evaluate include:

- Local and national trends in medical practices utilization.
- Technology changes and advances that may offer new services or change the way you provide your service (examples include laparoscopic surgery).
- General economic trends in your service area. For example, if you are in an area of economic decline with large facilities and employers closing down, you can assume that your practice is going to flatten, and you may even see decreases in revenue and volume in the coming year.
- Increased HMO activity and/or changes in health plan coverage by a dominant employer or a dominant insurer.

- Actions by competitors or new competitors entering the market, either in the form of group practices, more specialists, or actions taken by the hospital.
- Increasing use of capitation by health plans.

This is where the art of budget development comes into play. Again, I'm of the school where one is very conservative in projecting revenue. As noted earlier, if the numbers don't "feel right," then by all means adjust the numbers. Budgets are a forecast of the future, so by definition a budget will be wrong. In the end, management judgments must be made.

In developing revenue projections, practices can no longer simply multiply the utilization by the fee for each CPT code. The utilization attributable to capitation contracts must be pulled out of the equation before a fee-for-service computation can be made. The steps used to develop a revenue projection are as follows:

1. Develop the projected average number of members per month for each capitated contract. Multiply by the PMPY (per member per year) for each contract to develop the estimated annual revenue for each capitated contract.
2. Having identified fee-for-service revenue, multiply the projected utilization by CPT code by your fee. Important: Adjust the projected revenue by your collection rate (fee for service only) to determine a realistic projected revenue.
3. Adjust further by any risk pool/withhold contracts (how much of the withhold can you conservatively expect to see paid out to you, and when?).
4. Adding all these together, you have developed a projected revenue for the year.
5. Ask yourself: does this number seem realistic? Adjusting the projected revenue downward is a reasonable step if this is the judgment of the practice's management.

For the expense side of the budget, start with a list of your expenses per account with the year-to-date expense information (see Table 6–5). You will then want to trend the data to twelve

TABLE 6–5

Expense Budget Development Worksheet

Account	Year 1	Year 2	Difference	% Difference	Current YTD	Current Year 12 month Project	Difference	% Difference	Budget
Rent	2,000	2,100	100	5%	1,600	2,200	100	4.76%	2,300
Med suppl									
Salaries									
Total									

*YTD—Year to Date

months, which is admittedly not accurate because of the seasonality of some expenses as well as other factors. Finally, insert up to three years' worth of historic data, showing actual data and the year-to-year variance.

Some of the expense items are created from the data compiled in the schedules discussed earlier in this chapter. For the other items, you will need to make judgments, such as:

- Will our usage of medical supplies increase? Are there price increases expected?
- What will we budget for training? What are the major conferences for which we will send someone? Is the current budget sufficient?
- Are we planning significant one-time expenses for consultants? Special studies?
- Are we planning to recruit additional physicians or senior administrative staff? Have we allocated monies for recruitment advertisements, travel for interviews, and moving expenses?

And so on. In developing the budget, an excellent strategy is to bring the supervisors and managers into the process and let them help develop the budget line items, as they will be held responsible for and asked to maintain these items. Having some participation—even where the staff is overruled—goes a long way in educating the staff as to how the budget numbers have been arrived at. As a result, the staff is more likely to "buy in" to the budget that it has to administer.

The development of the budget takes place over two to three months, so circumstances and data availability (such as more current year-to-date information) changes over that time period. After the first draft has been compiled, the next stage involves analyzing and revising the expense budget to meet profit targets, changing circumstances, and environmental changes. This is also a time to include a contingency factor. The contingency factor represents 1 to 5 percent of the expense budget, and its purpose is to allow into the plan monies to account for unexpected expenses and changing circumstances. Again, since the purpose of a budget is to serve as a financial plan for the organization, having a contingency factor line is simply a means of insuring that sufficient resources will be set aside for the operation of the practice. It is not carte blanche to go out and spend it. However, it allows the practice managers to make decisions in the course of the year in conjunction with the board, knowing that the plan laid out will still be able to hold.

The last step of budget development involves finalizing the budget. This should be done no later than the last month of the year. Approval of the budget should be a function of the board of directors of the organization; this enables the management to ensure that the board (that is, the owners) have "signed on" in agreeing to the budget plan.

FINANCIAL STATEMENTS

Financial statements serve as a record of the financial performance of the organization—a recording of past actions that are the measure of the degree of success, as well as a basis for current and future decision making. There are many kinds of financial statements, each of which has a different purpose in providing information to management and/or other interested parties. The kinds of statements include:

- Profit and loss (aka revenue and expense).
- Comparison/variation of budget.
- Balance sheet.
- Cash position and cash flow.
- Audited and unaudited.
- Accrual versus cash basis.

The profit and loss, or revenue and expense, statement is the most common financial statement. The statement simply shows the revenue in, the expenses out, and the net result, which is the profit or excess revenue (or loss) remaining. The expenses can be booked on either a cash basis, which means that expenses are shown in total as cash is actually expensed and paid to a vendor, or on an accrual basis, which means that the expense is shown on the financial statement at the time the commitment for the expenditure is made. As an example, a pay period may end on the last day of the month and you will have an obligation to pay the payroll. On an accrual basis, you will show the payroll on the last day of the month. On a cash basis, however, you will show the payroll at the time you actually issue the paychecks. Expenses often will be shown higher on an accrual basis than on a cash basis, because there is a delay between the time the obligation is incurred and the time the cash is actually expended.

CHART OF ACCOUNTS

The purpose of a chart of accounts is to allocate expenses into categories based upon the kind of expense. This enables managers to determine how they are spending their money. The allocations are necessary for the costing of services and general management and control of the organization, as well as for tax purposes.

How this works is simple. Through a formal policy of the corporation, you establish the categories in a level of detail that meets your management needs. As an example, a small organization may simply have an account for insurance. Or you may split it out into a finer level of detail, listing life insurance, health insurance, and malpractice insurance, for example, as different accounts.

As a principle, all expenses must be allocated into an account when they are booked, either on an accrual or a cash basis. Although in your budget you will have a contingency line, this is not a valid account when it comes to booking expenses. It is appropriate to have an account titled "miscellaneous," but be careful about using this, as it should be used sparingly and only when the expense doesn't fit anywhere else. Ongoing expenses must have an account to call "home"; only a one-time or rare expense should be placed in the miscellaneous account.

When the accounts payable are being reviewed and prepared for payment, the assignment of the account can be made. Note that an invoice might be split among more than one account. As an example, a reimbursement for a conference may be split among:

- Conference / meeting / seminars.
- Books / journals (for books purchased at the conference exhibit hall).
- Marketing (taking a potential vendor or Medicare contractor to dinner).

Below is a sample chart of accounts. The Medical Group Management Association (MGMA) has a standard chart of accounts that provides an excellent base from which to develop your own. I do recommend that you develop your own, based upon MGMA's sample and the information in this book, and then review it with your outside accountant.

Sample Chart of Accounts (Expenses) for a Medical Practice

Accounting/legal

Fees paid for professional accounting, tax, and legal services.

Bank charges

Fees charged by banking institutions for services, including maintenance of accounts, credit card clearance, and such. Fees related to loans and supplies (checks, etc.) are charged to loan or office supply accounts.

Dues/books/journals

Membership dues in professional and business associations. Costs associated with the purchase of materials, books, and journals that are separate from membership dues but related to clinical and management subjects and materials for patient education and marketing are allocated to the appropriate accounts.

Consulting services

Professional fees and expenses for the use of outside consultants related to the management of the practice. Clinical services performed by nonemployees are charged under "purchased services."

Contributions

Donations made to charitable organizations not in connection with a marketing program.

Conventions/meetings/seminars

Registration fees and travel and miscellaneous expenses associated with out-of-town professional society meetings.

Equipment—Computer

Acquisition of computer hardware and network hardware and software.

Equipment—Medical

Equipment used for the diagnosis and treatment of patients.

Equipment—General

Purchase of machinery, office equipment, and testing and diagnostic equipment with a useful life of more than three years and a cost of more than $300.

Equipment/leases
Cost of monthly payment and repair of owned or leased equipment.

Furniture/fixtures
Movable items, including desks, chairs, exam tables, shelving, storage cabinets, walls, modular walls, and such.

Gifts
Presents to staff and others with a business connection to the practice.

Insurance—Business
Premium cost for business interruption and other general casualties.

Insurance—Property and casualty
Premium cost for property and casualty.

Insurance—Employee health
Premium for health insurance coverage for employees.

Insurance—Malpractice
Premium for professional liability coverage.

Insurance—Life and disability
Premium for life and disability insurance provided for employees.

Lab expenses
Supplies and minor equipment for clinical laboratory.

Laundry
Cost of cleaning uniforms, linens, and other washable material.

Leasehold improvements
Cost of building, installing, or changing the physical structure, including walls, doors, partitions (fixed or movable), signage, telephone hardware, electrical wiring, plumbing, and other utilities.

Licensee/permits
Cost of professional licenses, DEA permits, and business licenses and permits.

Maintenance and repairs
Ongoing care, cleaning, renovation, and repair of furniture, fixtures, and equipment, including painting, minor construction, preventative maintenance, and service calls for equipment.

Marketing expenses
Consultant fees, advertising, specialty products, health education brochures, and materials.

Medical supplies
Medical supplies and minor equipment used for day-to-day patient care.

Miscellaneous
Occasional, nonrecurring expenses that do not adequately fit into other categories.

Office expenses
Miscellaneous costs of running an office, including coffee/soda, storage, and newspapers and magazines for patients.

Office supplies/stationery
Stationery, pads, pens, forms, and minor office equipment.

Outside labor
Temporary, nonemployee workers.

Pension administration
Legal and management fees directly associated with the management of the pension fund.

Pension/staff
Contribution to the employee retirement fund.

Postage
Regular and express mail, other couriers, and express delivery services.

Recruitment expenses
Advertising, travel, entertainment, and relocation costs associated with the recruitment of new staff.

Rent
Cost of rented space.

Salaries/staff
Gross salaries paid to employees.

Salaries/technical
Salaries of technicians, nurses, and other nonphysician licensed professionals. (May be combined with salaries/staff.)

Salaries/physicians
Gross salaries of employee physician.

Taxes

Federal corporate
Federal income taxes paid on corporate earnings.

State corporate
State income taxes paid on corporate earnings.

Employment taxes
Employer portion of FICA (social security and medicare), and federal and state unemployment taxes.

Telephone
Cost of local and long distance service, pagers, and cellular phones, as well as maintenance of the internal phone system.

Training/education

Local seminars, courses, and meetings for staff.

Travel and entertainment

Business-related local travel, mileage, meals and entertainment.

Uniforms

Cost of uniforms and lab coats for physicians and staff.

REVENUE AND EXPENSE STATEMENT

The purpose of the revenue and expense statement is to present historical financial performance information for a defined period of time, typically a month, quarter, or year. These statements should be prepared at least monthly as a means of monitoring the practice's financial position.

Here's how it works:

On the revenue side, the statement will show in detail the cash collections or accrued revenue, typically by source, type of service, or third party payer (Table 6–6).

Both the revenue and the expense sides benefit from being measured against other's benchmarks. The most common measure is against budget, as seen in column D. A second common measure is against the same time period in the previous year. By measuring against the same time period, you can account for seasonal variations in your practice.

Since there are variations in practice volumes, practices need to look at patterns over time, such as by quarter. While we typically look at a quarter as the traditional three-month period (January to March, etc.), a "rolling" quarter presents you with current comparative data. A rolling quarter is the latest three-month period, whether or not it is a traditional quarter. In columns E and F above, the revenue and expense statement compares current activity by rolling quarter to the same rolling quarter in the previous year.

Column G above is a straight extrapolation of the year-to-date revenues to a 12-1 month, or one year, period. Obviously, it isn't until you get into the second half of the year that the extrapolation really gains some credibility, but it is easy to compute with a spreadsheet program and is worth looking over to spot any early warning signs.

TABLE 6–6

Format for Revenue Statement

A	B	C	D	E	F	G
Riverland Primary Care	**Current Month**	**Same Month Last Year**	**Variance to Budget**	**Change from Rolling Quarter**	**Change from Qtr Last Year**	**Year to Date**
Revenue:						
Medicare						
Medicaid						
HMO						
Commercial						
Total revenue						

The expense side of the revenue and expense statement shows the expenses for the period of time by each of the accounts, as outlined in the chart of accounts. The format is the same as that of the revenue side, as outlined above. As with the revenue side, you compare the monthly expenses with the same period last year and the current year rolling quarter with the same rolling quarter from the previous year.

The one number that can be computed at this point is the expense to revenue (E/R) ratio. The E/R ratio presents expenses as a percentage of collected revenue. It is a critical indicator of the overhead and operating costs of the practice and is a determinant of profitability. While there are varying opinions as to what the E/R ratio should be, this is one of those numbers that is most relevant in relation to itself. By tracking it over time, you can see how your E/R ratio changes. It will fluctuate month to month. Long-term, quarterly, semiannual, and annual numbers are really the better indicator of how your E/R ratio is trending.

The net difference between the revenue and expenses, as noted earlier, is the ADI—available for distribution and investment. The revenue and expense statement (Table 6–7) also can show the collection ratio, which is a critical indicator of the success of the collection effort and the reasonableness of the fees versus the actual payments. The collection ratio is expressed as a percentage, representing the cash collections as a percentage of gross billings. I have experienced a collection ratio of over 100 percent in a month where billings was down but a whole lot of back due monies were paid to the practice.

ACCOUNTS PAYABLE SCHEDULE

Accounts payable represent the compilation of the invoices and bills that the practice is obligated to pay at a given period of time. The accounts payable schedule is a management tool that is maintained on an ongoing basis, presenting for management a current listing of outstanding obligations and when payment is required.

Here's how an accounts payable schedule works. All invoices are entered into accounts payable files as they are received. Many computer systems can handle this automatically; at the very least, it can be done on a manual ledger. Noninvoiced, that is, recurring

TABLE 6–7

Format for Revenue and Expense Statement

A	B	C	D	E	F	G
Riverland Primary Care (date)	**Current Month**	**Same Month Last Year**	**Variance to Budget**	**Rolling Quarter**	**Change from Qtr Last Year**	**Year to Date**
Revenue:						
Medicare						
Medicaid						
HMO						
Commercial						
Total revenue						
Expense:						
Salaries						
General insurance						
Rent						
Equipment leases						
Travel						
Medical supplies						
Books/journals						
Miscellaneous						
Total expenses						
ADI:						
Collection rate:						

TABLE 6–8

Aged Accounts Payable Schedule

Riverland Medical Practice
Schedule of Aged Accounts Payable
As of: October 31, 1996

Vendor	Current < 30 Days	30–60 Days	60–90 Days	> 90 Days	Total
E&A Real Estate Management Co.	$1,000				$1,000
Andrew Medical Supply	$345	$565			$910
Lawrence Law Firm			$135		$135
Chuck's Insurance		$2,345			$2,345
Bill's Subscription Service		$45	$65		$110
Total	**$1,345**	**$2,955**	**$200**		**$4,500**

obligations such as rent, lease payments, and the like also are logged. These items are ones where there is a monthly obligation or a more frequent obligation to make a payment, although there may be no formal notice sent to the practice. Mortgages and loans, for example, may have a coupon book issued that is to be used for payments. By developing and maintaining this schedule, the practice will have a running compilation of its obligations.

The schedule shown in Table 6–8 example is what is called an "aged" schedule. Much like accounts receivable records, payables are aged in relation to the payment due date. Current payables are those that, although not yet paid, still have less than 30 days past the due date. As you can see, the dollars owed to each vendor are listed in the proper aging column, even if one vendor may have multiple invoices that are due with different ages.

The accounts payable schedule should be allocated by age, that is, as follows:

- Current—less than 30 days have elapsed from the due date.
- 30, 60, 90, or more days past due.

As bills age, some vendors may start imposing late fees and charging interest. Pay attention to late fees, as some vendors (such as utilities) can or will cut off service to you. Others can report your payment history and impact your credit standing. Additionally, many of the vendors you work with are small companies, often smaller than your practice. If for no other reason than an ethical one, paying the "smaller" guys promptly helps them and earns good will in the community. As a rough guide, stay within 30 to 45 days current on your payables as a good management practice.

In making your weekly payables budget, use the aged accounts payable schedule as your basis. You will always want to pay obligations that are routine and due every month, such as utilities. Once you fall behind on these expenses, the next bill is rolling in. It is especially important that insurance premiums are paid on time; otherwise, you may find that the policy has been canceled.

A good way to plan and budget for payables is to print out the aged report two to three days before you plan to mail the checks. Identify those bills that must be paid, as discussed above. Then look to the oldest payables and work toward the current payables in making your selections. If you have built up large obligations with a vendor, it will prefer that you clear up the oldest amounts due first, since this improves its financial statement. Old accounts receivable are not viewed well by lenders and bankers, who may discount them in assessing creditworthiness.

A final suggestion: if you can't afford to pay all of the monies owed to a vendor, a partial payment is at least some evidence of good faith. It is important that the vendor be called and the situation discussed honestly; don't make payment promises you may not be able to keep. However, a promise to call the vendor as your situation changes and to send monies along the way will enhance your credibility and help you through a difficult time. This is not a tactic to simply delay paying someone, for, like the little boy who cried "wolf," eventually your reputation will be tarnished and you will find yourself either cut off or dealt with on a cash on delivery (COD) basis.

ACCOUNTS RECEIVABLE

Your accounts receivable (A/R) represent uncollected cash. As such, they are an asset of the organization. Rising A/R are a warning sign of a problem in the practice. In and of itself, however, the A/R figure is mostly a number relevant to itself. The A/R for a practice can be expressed in one of two ways: (1) as a dollar amount, or (2) in terms of the number of days of service represented.

Under capitation arrangements, your A/R should be minimal, as you should be receiving your payment every month on time and your copayments at the time of service.

To control your A/R, reports should be run on a monthly basis and a review should be conducted on outstanding A/R based upon days outstanding (in other words, greater than 30, 60, 90, and 120 days). As discussed earlier, bill promptly, electronically, and often. After 30 days for electronic claims and 45 days for paper claims, any outstanding claims should be rebilled. Once a receivable goes beyond 90 days, the chances of recovery drop off dramatically, particularly if you are looking for payment from an individual patient.

Many third party payers also place timeframes within which claims must be filed. There also are varying time restrictions in how far back you can go to submit or resubmit a claim. As with many business and customer relationships, phone calls often go a long way to prodding patients and carriers toward making a payment.

The insurance claim inquiry form, shown in Figure 6–2 that follows is one means of following up an overdue receivables. Basically, you need to always document any follow-up efforts. If you call the carrier, document who made the call, the time, who you spoke with, and what happened. Be wary of taping calls. Although it may be legal, you probably will need to notify the other party that you are doing so. The carrier also may be notifying you that it is taping the conversation.

Another frequent measure of A/R is the "number of days in receivable." Since A/R represent charges for services rendered that have yet to be paid, the total A/R due represents the sum of many days' worth of services.

FIGURE 6–2

Insurance Claim Inquiry Form

Ashley Cooper Medical Associates
911 Medical Way
Folly Beach, SC 29306
(803) 555-3232

Insurance Inquiry Form

Insurance Company: ______________________

Address: ______________________

Patient's Name: ______________ Cert. No. ______________

Address: ______________________

Group No. ______________________

Date of Service	Procedure Code	Charge	Paid Date	Patient Acct. No.

Question: ______________________

____

Provider No. ______________ Provider Name ______________

Answer: ______________________

____

Provider Services Rep: __________ Phone No. ______________

Name of Person Calling ______________ Date ________ Time of Call: ________

____
Signature

To compute your days' outstanding in accounts receivable:

1. Take your current A/R number.
2. Divide by your annualized total billings.
3. Multiply the ratio (see step [2]) by 360 days.
4. The result is the number of days in A/R.

As an example, if your current A/R is $300,000 and your billings annualized to 12 months total $900,000, that equals one-third. Multiply one-third by 360, and the result is 120, meaning that the A/R is 120 days. That means 120 days of service rendered are due to you as uncollected cash.

Gaining control of the finances of a practices is the critical step to gaining control of the practice. Many a physician loses sleep because they feel that their practice is "out of control." What is missing is a portrait of the practice, including a systematic mechanism that provides data and information on the financial state of the practice.

It will take time to build the schedules and reports presented in this chapter, but once built, they are fairly easy to maintain on a monthly basis. Direct your staff to make the preparation of financial report the priority at the beginning of each month. Management must then review these reports, ask questions, and get any clarifications. This way, management clearly conveys the message that finances and financial reporting are very important.

As you do this, use your accountant as a sounding board and advisor. Much of the information that will be collected will also be needed by the accountant for tax filing purposes, so it will make everyone's life easier if the data is collected and formatted the first time around. A good accountant will also help you institute the proper controls within your system to insure accuracy and accountability.

7 CHAPTER

Cost Management

Up until now, our discussion has focused on the revenue-generating side of the business equation. A business grows and thrives by focusing its efforts on growing the size of its revenue, maximizing revenue for every person and every dollar in costs. That said, the cost side can sneak up on many practices and cause serious damage and havoc before the crisis is back under control or the physicians are forced into a fire sale to a hospital or physician practice management company.

Medical practices are facing a world where revenue is decreasing and fixed in advance. As revenue becomes increasingly fixed and predictable, the critical success factor is shifted toward the ability to control costs in relation to revenue—in other words, profit.

For health care organizations, the "traditional" estimate has been that 60 to 70 percent of an organization's expenses goes to employee salaries and benefits. Since the physician, a licensed practitioner, is the principal generator of revenue, the only way to increase revenue is for the physician to see more patients or perform more services per hour. Using the ancillary staff the physician's time can be leveraged by performing more services that require the presence of a physician in the office, even though she is not the one who is actually going to perform the test. Examples of this are lab work, certain radiology exams, nuclear imaging, and stress tests.

Another way for practices to maximize revenue per hour is through the use of midlevel practitioners, such as physician assistants, nurse practitioners, and nurse midwives. These midlevel practitioners are of most value and have the most experience in primary care settings. When I take my child to the pediatrician with a possible ear infection, in reality I do not need a board certified pediatrician with subspecialty training in neonatology to look in my child's ears and determine, "Yep, they're red." Even when the physician is not present in the office, midlevel practitioners can be seeing patients, billing, making hospital rounds, assisting with some of the back paperwork, answering patient calls, and the like.

COSTING SERVICES

The perennial question facing health care organizations is: what does it cost to provide our services? By and large, cost accounting in health care is still in its infancy, as providers struggle with mountains of data, but little usable information and few standards for establishing costs. As has been noted several times in this book, as revenues both decrease and are increasingly fixed in advance, it is the management of costs, rather than the generation of revenue, which needs to become the focus of management attention.

Medical practices, fortunately, have a relatively easy way to compute the costs of their services. The relative value units (RVU) system—so feared and hated when first implemented by Medicare—conveniently establishes a common means of measuring the resources consumed (the costs) for each common procedure terminology (CPT) code.

As discussed earlier, the full name for this system is the resource based relative value units system (RBRVU). The underlying thesis is that it establishes a uniform means of measuring the practice expense, malpractice expense, and work effort that goes into the delivery of each service represented by a CPT code. The RVU for each code, then, represents the amount of resources consumed relative to the amount of resources consumed by another CPT code. As an example, the RVU for code 99213 (Office or other outpatient visit—established patient) is .96. The value for the professional component of a coronary artery bypass surgery (code 33510) is 58.04.

In measuring the cost of a service, what is being measured are the resources consumed. There are four types of resources in any organization:

1. Human (your staff).
2. Physical (facilities and equipment).
3. Financial (cash and other financial needs).
4. Information and technology (information gathering and processing systems and technology aids).

The resources and costs of any organization can be placed in one of these four categories. The work done over the years in the various RBRVU systems, culminating with the Harvard study used by Medicare, has been based upon surveys and on-site studies of the costs inherent in running a physician practice. The values have some updates every year, and the HCFA currently is studying the entire system and looking toward a major review in 1997, five years after Medicare instituted the system for setting the Medicare fee schedule.

Just as we establish a conversion factor (CF) to establish the fee, we can use the RVU system to establish the cost per CPT code. This can be accomplished by following the steps below.

1. Compute the total expenses of the practice, using either the previous year or the last full 12-month period. In doing so, we immediately run into a problem, however. The question now confronts us: What's an expense? Specifically, how do we treat the monies paid to the physicians?

My recommendation is that the salaries, bonuses, and benefits paid to the employee physicians (physicians who are not owners of the practice as shareholders or partners) be counted as an expense. Any monies that are fundamentally dividends for shares or otherwise paid to owners should not be counted. What is to be counted are those dollars that are obligations of the practice, regardless of the profitability of the practice. Salaries to employees are obligations, but dividends or other distributions of profits are not, as they are paid only if there is a profit and will vary depending upon the size of the profit.

2. Compute the total number of RVUs delivered in the year (see page 103 for a detailed description of how to do this).

TABLE 7-1

Cost Computation Procedure

Riverland Primary Care Group
Cost per RVU Computation
For Calendar Year 1996
9/30/95

CPT Code #	RBRVU	1995 Proj. Util.	Total RVUs	Expense Conv. Factor	Cost Per CPT code	Fee	Profit/ Loss
99201	0.83	150	125	$58.12	**$48.24**	$38.00	($10.24)
99202	1.31	125	164	$58.12	**$76.14**	$75.00	($1.14)
99203	1.77	300	531	$58.12	**$102.87**	$125.00	$22.13
99204	2.59	335	868	$58.12	**$150.53**	$214.00	$63.47
99205	3.22	200	644	$58.12	**$187.15**	$250.00	$62.85
Total		**1,110**	**2,331**				
Total Expenses: $135,475							

Steps:

1. Total practice expenses for the year ($135,475)
2. Divided by total practice RVUs for the year (2,331)
3. Equal Conversion factor per RVU for practice expenses: $58.12
4. Multiply Expense Conversion Factor by RVU for each code to determine cost per CPT code
5. Subtract cost from fee to determine profit/loss for each code

TABLE 7-2

Service Profitability Analysis

CPT Code	Description	RVU	PECF	Cost	Revenue	Profit/Loss
99201	Office visit	.83	$25.00	$20.75	$29.88	$9.13
93000	EKG	.80	$25.00	$20.00	$28.80	$8.80
Total		1.63		$40.75	$58.68	$15.93

3. Divide the total expenses by the total RVUs to determine the dollar expense per relative value unit: the practice expense conversion factor (PECF).

4. Multiply the PECF by the RVU for each code, and the result is the practice cost per CPT code (PCC)

Now that the cost per CPT code has been determined, you now can evaluate your costs and profitability using various parameters.

1. For each CPT code, compare the PCC to the fee paid to determine your profit or loss per code.
2. Look at your key services and compile the multiple codes for the services to determine your cost, revenue, and profit or loss. In Table 7-2, a simple example of this analysis is presented.

The drawback of the RVU-based cost accounting system is that it is specific neither to the practice nor a specialty. RVUs were developed from a national study. Since RVUs are used by all specialties providing the same coded service, it does not account for variations in the services provided by one specialty as opposed to another.

Cost accounting is, in itself, a potentially complicated subject area that is already the subject of complete texts and college courses (and a business network program), which is why I find the RVU-based system so appealing. With any cost accounting system, there are certain assumptions that need to be made:

- What are the services to cost?
- What are the direct costs?
- What are the indirect costs?
- On what basis are indirect costs allocated?

I've gone through the exercise of costing services in a practice using a cost allocation methodology, and it's not a pretty sight. Since the allocation of indirect costs is somewhat of a subjective decision, the methodology used is then subject to dispute and attack. There are a number of resources available that can further assist you in costing services, including several from the Medical Group Management Association (MGMA).

There are several other ways to look at the costs of services that are related directly to how managed care plans pay for services. In capitation-related methodologies, services are costed and paid for as an average for all patients. Rather than being paid a different fee for each service, the flat rate is being paid to cover all services. Revenue, then, must exceed the average cost in order to be profitable. Examples of this include average cost per patient and average cost per encounter.

The average cost per patient method of costing services involves the following steps:

1. Determine the total practice expenses (less owner compensation).
2. Determine the number of unique patients seen by the practice in the year. (A unique patient is an individual patient, regardless of the number of services provided.)
3. Divide step (1) by step (2) to reach the average cost per patient.
4. Identify all revenue from an HMO.
5. Identify the number of unique patients in that HMO.
6. Divide step (4) by step (5) to reach the average revenue per HMO patient.
7. Compare steps (3) and (5) to determine the average cost for the HMO patient with the average revenue for the HMO patient and identify the percentage profit margin.

The average cost per encounter method of costing services, on the other hand, involves the following steps:

1. Determine the total expenses for the practice (less owner compensation).

2. Determine the number of physician encounters for the year (including all physician services, regardless of location—hospital, office, etc.).
3. Divide step (1) by step (2) to identify the average cost per physician encounter.
4. Identify physician encounters for HMO patients.
5. Identify the total revenue for the HMO.
6. Divide step (5) by step (4) to identify the average revenue per physician encounter.
7. Compare steps (3) and (6) and identify the percentage profit margin.

Encounter-based comparisons are obviously a fuzzy number, since all encounters are not created equal. For example, an encounter that is a hospital visit is different from an encounter that is an office visit. This does provide yet another piece of information in the puzzle.

COST REDUCTION STRATEGIES

For most businesses, the best way to lower the ratio of expenses to revenues is to increase revenues, that is, garner the advantages of marginal costs. For medical practices, however, we face an environment of flat or potentially declining revenue. Maintaining and increasing profits, therefore, is dependent upon the ability to garner improved returns on revenue, that is, return on a per-unit basis. This is accomplished by the ability to lower overhead and operating expenses and reengineer business processes to maximize productivity—services per person, per hour, and such.

The first area to tackle is the obvious: can expenses be reduced or can further benefits, or value per dollar, be realized from the expenses? Some of the areas where cost reductions can take place have to do with the usage and scheduling of staff. Unless a practice is principally office-based, there will be blocks of time when patients are not being scheduled. Therefore, part-time staff might be used only during office hours to help move patients through. Obviously, you still need staff for the constant flow of work and phone calls coming in through the course of a day.

Preparation time also is necessary, pulling charts, reviewing charts, looking for referrals, making sure lab work has been done, and so on. These tasks do require a full-time staff member, for continuity purposes, as well.

The contribution of the staff to the practice is not only a function of the number of full time equivalents, but also a function of the mix of different skills. You can divide your staff into five tiers of skills based upon the degree of training and specialized skill, as follows:

- Level 5: Practitioners, such as physicians assistants, midwives and physical therapists.
- Level 4: Technical staff, such as radiology technicians.
- Level 3: Medically-skilled staff, such as medical assistants.
- Level 2: Secretarial, such as transcriptionists and executive secretaries.
- Level 1: Clerical, such as receptionists, schedulers, and clerical support.

By restructuring the mix of your employees, you also can maximize the productivity and benefits from the dollars invested in the staff.

Other areas of possible cost reduction include liability policies and health insurance, which we will discuss next.

With regard to liability policies, every couple of years it is worth reevaluating your property and casualty insurance. It is also an excellent idea to make sure that your coverage is sufficient to cover your practice's needs. An easy way to assist yourself is to make a videotape walking through your office, room by room, with commentary on what the different equipment is. A copy of this tape can be given to your agent, accountant, or other business advisor to keep off site. In the event of a disaster (i.e., a loss), you then have the best documentation of your practice in your possession. In addition to this, you should possess business interruption insurance. I know of at least two practices that suffered fires which basically wiped out all of the medical records. Business interruption insurance covers many of the costs incurred until you are able to reopen your practice after a disaster, including: staff costs, locating and moving to a new location (even a temporary one), reconstructing medical records, acquiring replacement software and computers, and such. This brings up the point of backing up your computer system daily and moving diskettes or tapes to an off-site location. Internally, records—particularly diskettes, tapes, or computer-based records—can be kept in fireproof safes that can be purchased fairly inexpensively.

Worker's comp is another area always worth taking a look at, particularly if you have a history of claims against you. Also, as your practice gets larger, you are more likely to be able to enter into a pool where pricing is not community-rated but is practice-specific.

Regarding the reduction of costs related to health insurance, if you want to reduce your employee health insurance expense, consider mandating an HMO. You will find that managed care organization pricing can be significantly less than your standard indemnity plan. However, unless your practice is big enough, you will not have a sufficient number of employees to offer two plans.

Employees are used to the idea that managed care organizations are being required and mandated by more and more employers. One other way to control costs is by premium sharing, whereby your employees are asked to pay typically between 5 percent and 10 percent of the cost of the premium. This also will force off of your plan those who are part of a dual wage earner family and may be carrying two health insurance policies. It is very common for small businesses to pay for the cost of health insurance for an employee but impose the copremium payment, if not 100 percent of the premium payment, on the family plans. Given the fact that many practices are staffed by women, and in many areas a preponderance of single mothers, you may want to carefully consider this alternative: this benefit may be worth a great deal, both in terms of dollars and goodwill to your staff. By all means, however, unless prohibited by the insurance carriers, it is terrible public relations and bad form for a physician's office not to be providing health insurance coverage for its employees. I have, however, seen that, even in some fairly large practices.

You can trim a few dollars and provide a valuable benefit to your employees by setting up a Section 125 plan, named after the section of The Internal Revenue Code. A payroll service, or maybe your accountant, can handle this for a one-time set-up fee of several hundred dollars. This section of the Code allows deductions for the coinsurance payments for health insurance and certain other types of benefits to be deducted before taxes from the employee's check. In other words, there are no income taxes paid on it by the employee. At the same time, the employer is relieved of paying Social Security taxes on these dollars, saving you some money right there. It is a nice benefit that goes a long way in terms of putting money in your employees' pockets. It also enables you to look at offering group health and disability on a pretax, payroll deduction basis. Again, this is a benefit that can engender goodwill among your employees, enable you to buy in to a similar kind of policy on top of any individual policies you might have, and lower your costs. There are limitations as to what carriers will write in terms of personal disability policies on an individual. A group policy is one way to add to your coverage for minimal—and in some cases actually no cost.

Group purchasing organizations have been around for a long time and are very popular among hospitals. You may be able to access some of the large ones, such as Voluntary Hospitals of America (VHA) and the Premier/American Health Systems/Sun Health Network (now called simply Premier). In addition, MGMA offers a group purchasing program as well. These programs work by negotiating large contracts with national organizations, thus gaining significant discounts and prices. As a participant, you pay an administrative fee to the group purchasing organization. For larger practices, as you get bigger, your practice will have sufficient volume that your savings will begin to outweigh the costs of belonging to the plan.

In addition to liability policies and health insurance, other cost savings can be achieved on a smaller scale. For example, office supplies have basically now been driven to pricing levels governed by the large office warehouse stores, such as Office Depot, Office Max, Staples, and the like. Nevertheless, it is always worth shopping, and there are some national mail-order supply companies such as Viking, Quill, and others if your market area does not have competitive pricing.

Phone service is another area always to watch. With the new telecommunications bills and competition in the local and long distance markets now, it behooves you to keep an eye on the various deals being offered to businesses. I am not a proponent of frequent changes in phone service, since phone service is the lifeline of your business. However, it is worth watching for competitive deals.

Certain management functions for small practices are frequently contracted out, such as the preparation of financial statements and compilations, billing, and bookkeeping services. These services are worth pricing, and it also may be worth bringing some of these functions in-house as you grow. New computer software makes many of these functions a lot easier and cheaper to perform. However, I am an advocate of hiring a payroll service to perform the payroll function. Payroll services are amazingly efficient at producing payroll checks. They also can handle the electronic deposit of checks, which is a very nice benefit for your employees and yourself. It may make sense to contract for billing services, although you will need to be very careful about the quality of the work performed.

Legal and accounting services are worth taking a look at by placing a retainer. Look at the volume of dollars being spent on these services and the kinds of services you are buying. Repetitive services, such as compilations, financial statement preparation, and perhaps even tax returns, are worth locking down a fixed monthly price. Attorneys and accountants are familiar with retainer arrangements and you can discuss this with them.

Retirement management investment services are a hotbed of competition. Again, my personal advice is that stability is valuable. Making frequent changes in your investment management is not a good idea. However, it is worth looking at historical returns and, more importantly, the quality of the advice and management services you get. Also, consider whether any fees are being charged by the management company itself above and beyond whatever fee is being charged for direct brokerage services and by the mutual funds themselves. Every company will tell you that is has a better deal, that it has someone who outperformed the market the previous year, but, as is fairly commonly known, few are able to claim that year after year, and your retirement money should not be placed completely at risk. The key to retirement investment management is allocating your assets in different levels of risk, depending upon your personal values and what you are comfortable with, as well as where you are in your life cycle.

If healthcare operated under the "normal" patterns of economic behavior, the emphasis would be on increasing revenue rather than reducing costs. Since practices are faced with revenues that may be flat or decreasing, cost does become a major concern. From a management perspective, then, the key is value: maximizing revenue for every dollar in expense. The areas discussed in this chapter are but some of the many steps in achieving that goal.

8 CHAPTER

Strategic Issues

Until now, I've focused on the "micro" issues of creating and managing change in the medical practice. Many physicians have responded to the pressures of the new realities in health care by retiring, moving, or turning the keys over to a management company or a hospital. Avoidance is an honorable, time-honored strategy. Medical practices today are facing their most difficult and stressful times; in fact, their very existence is threatened. Make no mistake, however. It is very much a part of the business revolution shaking our world economy to its core.

Historically, medical practices have operated as a cottage industry, that is, many small businesses make up the marketplace. In the 1980s and 1990s, the industry experienced very rapid growth in terms of revenue and profits. This was driven by changes in Medicare reimbursement, which actually profited many hospitals, and the growth of an aging population in need of and demanding more and more services. This kind of growth attracted professional investment and venture capital money, which flowed into a flood of companies serving the health care marketplace. Some of these companies, such as Columbia/HCA, Medical Care International, MedPartners, Caremark, and the like were predicated on the idea that by bringing together a diverse group of small companies, consolidating back office functions, and bringing in professional management, they can leverage economies of scale into more efficient, lower cost operations that also will be more profitable for all concerned. This conviction, coupled with the very strong push from employers to lower health care costs, set up the revolution and upheaval we are experiencing today in the organization, finance, and delivery of health care services.

The first decision that a medical practice must make is whether or not to affiliate with other health care organizations. Then it must determine the degree of integration that it is comfortable with.

Figure 8-1 presents the principal options that confront a medical practice. As with many things in health care, the names may change, but the culprits are still the same.

The first critical decision is to decide whether the physicians prefer to remain autonomous or if they prefer to affiliate through some level of integration with other practices and/or providers. By remaining autonomous, the practice may still seek out managed care contracts or even join a captive independent practice association (IPA) in order to contract with a particular health maintenance organization (HMO), but it may not choose to join any other joint venture or cooperative enterprise.

A decision to pursue integration is one decision, but it is the *degree* of integration that first confronts the medical practice with a decision that sits at the core strategy of the organization. In all, a medical practice faces three options:

1. Contract for all management services.
2. Join a network of independent practices.
3. Consolidate with one or more practices into a group.

However, there is a fourth option that is becoming increasing popular: sell the practice and become an employee or independent contractor of the new "owner," which may be a hospital or physician practice management company.

Autonomy presents its own set of risks and rewards; the reward is embodied in the continued freedom and control of one's destiny that comes with owning one's own business, yet the risk lies in not being able to compete in the "new health care realities." Even practices that choose to remain autonomous face yet another decision point—whether or not to expand by adding additional physicians and/or offices.

FIGURE 8-1

Medical Practice Integration Decision Tree

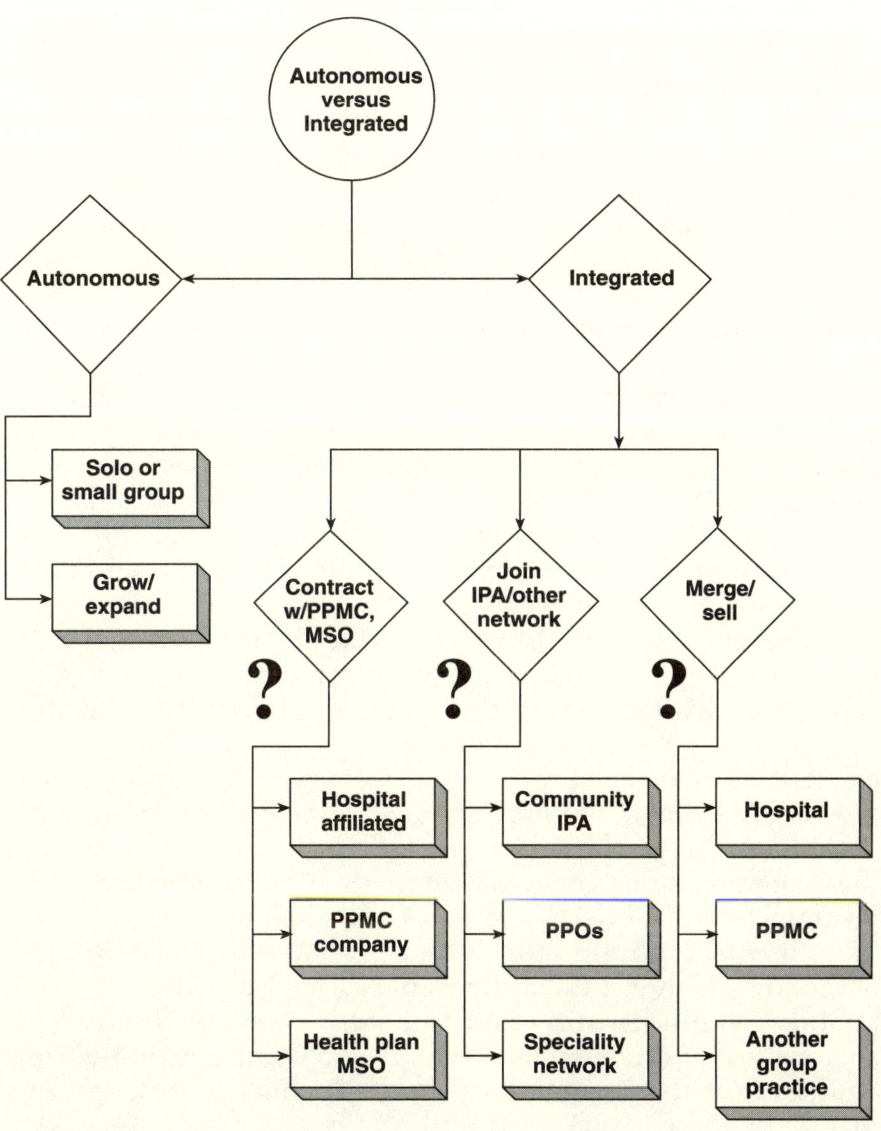

STAGES OF PHYSICIAN PRACTICE INTEGRATION

There are about seven stages of physician practice integration. The least integrated model is the solo practitioner. Next up on the scale is what is known as a group without walls, or GWW. A group without walls is a group practice that operates using multiple sites. As a first step, several small solo practitioners will band together into one entity but continue to operate in their old locations. This is often the case where the solo practitioners own their individual buildings, have leases in place, and the like.

The next stage up is the group practice, which may or may not occupy one locale. In this case, however, the real estate involved is more a function of the needs of the entire group rather than the historical needs of the group's members.

The next step up is what is known as a contracting network, called an independent practice association, or IPA. While some HMOs have developed IPAs for contracting purposes, there are a number of IPAs around the country that are banding together of a number of groups and solo physicians into a corporate organization. This IPA then in turn can enter into contracts with HMOs and other employers directly.

The next stage in physician practice integration is the physician hospital integration. Most commonly, this takes the form of a physician–hospital organization, or PHO. Readers who have been around a while may be familiar with the old concept of medical staff hospital (MeSH) organizations. The idea behind MeSH organizations, as with PHOs, was to align the interests of the physicians and the hospitals. Unfortunately, these organizations chose to reflect the 1980s mentality of the fast buck and the big hit and focused a great deal on real estate investments, building office buildings, investing in MRIs and other high technology equipment, as well as other assorted business ventures unrelated to health care. As we are well aware, most of these failed miserably and other consulting firms had to repair the damage done by the original consulting firms that set up these MeSH organizations.

PHOs, on the other hand, appear to have actually lived up to some of their billing in a number of cases and are evolving out of their initial rationale. PHOs have tended to focus on the healthcare arena, beginning with their effective formation of an IPA organization that includes a hospital that goes out and bids for contracts with managed care organizations (MCOs). MCOs, as you are aware, need both the physician network as well as the hospital in order to provide services to their members.

Some PHOs now have evolved into taking on management functions by either buying practice assets or providing management services in the contract to members of the PHO.

The next level of integration is when the practice integrates with another management company or with a payer. Management companies, to be discussed in detail later, will typically acquire the assets of a practice and contract with the physicians to provide the management services. Some payers, such as Blue Cross Western Pennsylvania, Aetna, and Prudential, either own practices outright or have long-term contracts with specific physician groups in order to provide primary care, and in some cases specialty care, services for their members.

The highest level of integration is the integrated delivery system, or IDS. A true integrated system combines all the provider components, including a network of hospitals in a geographic area (including a tertiary care hospital), specialty and primary care physicians, dental services, mental health, rehab and so on. In short, the idea is to provide one-stop shopping for a managed care organization. The IDS also is an ideal vehicle for assuming a global or full risk capitation contract. Since the IDS owns or controls all of the provider pieces, it can allocate dollars among the pieces in a manner that will best serve the common needs of the system as a whole. The IDS has the capability, as well, to develop its own HMO product and/or contract directly with employers and employer groups, using either a fee-for-service or a risk-based model.

LEGAL ISSUES IN INTEGRATION

There are a number of common legal issues that arise as physicians integrate, such as:

- Fraud and abuse.
- Antitrust.

- Corporate practice of medicine.
- Tax-exempt status.
- Employee benefit plans.

Let's consider these one by one.

Fraud and Abuse

There are a host of business practices that are perfectly legal in most sectors of the economy but, if undertaken by a physician group when dealing with Medicare, would fall under the fraud and abuse sections of the Medicare/Medicaid statutes and possibly constitute a felony under federal law. The principal example of this has to do with any compensation that can be construed to have been paid or made in return for a referral. Baxter's former Caremark subsidiary provides one of the classic examples of an ongoing fraud; this has been settled only recently, after Caremark was spun off by Baxter as an independent company. Regulations have been issued to implement the so-called "Stark" amendments (named for the California Congressman) which present those activities which are banned and those which are covered by a "safe harbor" provision and would generally be considered permissible. Examples of business practices that these regulation construe as fraud and abuse include: below market rents for office space; management and training of staff; and the provision of management services, such as billing services at below market rates.

Antitrust

Because medical practices are considered independent businesses, any grouping of medical practices that discusses and agrees upon its fees to be charged, conspires not to negotiate with HMO plans, or otherwise engages in anticompetitive practices potentially violates the antitrust laws. The example of sharing or agreeing on fee schedules to be charged is considered price fixing. The agreement not to negotiate with HMOs would be considered restraint of trade.

The most famous case of price fixing occurred in Maricopa County outside of Phoenix, Arizona, where there was an agreement as to the maximum fee schedule among the members of a medical foundation. There has also been a case involving an association of varied dentists who negotiated and bargained a price on behalf of its members. And, finally, a group of anesthesiologists once conspired to reject the reimbursement levels proposed by a Blue Cross plan. Essentially, a group of competitors cannot conspire to refuse to do business with an insurer, such as refusing to sign on with an HMO. In a recent case in New York's Long Island area, seven hospitals conspired to agree that no one hospital would sign a contract with an HMO without the consent of the other hospitals. The hospitals settled this matter out of court to "avoid the cost of litigation." As a mildly aware observer would realize, of course, these hospitals were caught red-handed. In a nutshell, don't do it! Many of the Medical Group Management Association (MGMA) meetings now start with a declaration that no discussion of fees can occur in the course of the meeting because of the obvious danger that, should one practice identify its pricing, it may be copied by others.

The other antitrust violation that practices have to be aware of is monopolization or domination of the marketplace. This can occur when a sufficient number of specialists or primary care physicians in a market area (i.e., enough to be able to artificially raise prices) band together in a group. This consolidation of the market may not be allowed by the Justice Department. Consolidations should be reviewed with your counsel because an antitrust review is driven by the specific circumstances of the proposed transaction and, therefore, it is not possible to give clear rules and advice within this book.

In August, 1996, the Federal Trade Commission (FIC) and the U.S. Department of Justice issued the document, "Revised Policy Statements on Health Care Antitrust Enforcement." The document, in full, is available on paper through either department, or over the Internet at the FTC's web site, (see appendix F). Specifically, the policy statement establishes "antitrust safety zones," which describe conduct that, absent extraordinary circumstances, the department will not challenge. The statement expands the types of situations in which physician networks are allowed. These situations include those where determining whether or not to allow a proposed arrangement depends upon whether the impact of the procompetitive behavior is greater than the impact of the anticompetitive behavior. The statement makes very clear that the objective is not to define the boundaries of allowable conduct, but rather, to describe safety zone conduct and provide additional guidance as to where certain conduct will still be allowed, even if it falls outside the safety zones.

Corporate Practice of Medicine

In most states the only parties who may be owners of a professional practice such as a physician practice are licensed members of the profession. Some states will allow hospitals and HMOs to employ physicians because of the granting of a license by the state. Many states, however, forbid this. This falls under the provision except commonly known as the Corporate Practice of Medicine Act, whereby a corporation—except a professional corporation—cannot employ professionals to practice their profession.

When the physician practice management companies such as MedPartners and Phycor "acquire" a practice, what they actually do is acquire the assets of a practice and contract with the remaining physician corporation to provide their services for the physicians. The remaining physician corporation may no longer hold any assets or perform any functions other than employing the physicians.

Tax Exempt Status

In order for a tax-exempt hospital to maintain its tax exempt status, it must be operated for the benefit of the community and there may be no personal gain or sharing of excess revenue or profits by individuals. When hospitals acquire a physician practice, however, there are two concerns: (1) is the price paid for the practice reflective of fair market values, and (2) a portion of the profits from the practice are paid to the physician. Physicians are allowed to be paid a fair market wage and they may also receive bonuses based upon specific performance criteria. Again, this is an area that may need to be reviewed with your outside counsel or your accountant. Be aware that a number of states and localities have endeavored to levy property and business taxes on what are legally tax-exempt organizations under the grounds of state law; others have tried to levy their business license tax on the "for-profit" operations of a not-for-profit organization. Owning and operating medical practices is one way for a municipality to attack a hospital's not-for-profit status, because the hospital is engaging in what is principally a for-profit activity.

Employee Benefit Plans

Because of the Employee Retirement and Income Security Act (ERISA), employee benefit plans, particularly retirement plans, are subject to very close scrutiny by the U.S. Labor Department and the Internal Revenue Service. Breaking up a plan, closing down a plan, or merging a plan with the plan of another organization after several practices have merged all are subject to complex rules. Again, outside counsel with expertise in these areas needs to be consulted to make sure these plans are done by the book. You otherwise are at risk of losing your tax exempt deductions for your contributions in the plan, and of course, at risk of incurring fines.

Elements of a Group Practice

When it comes to the merger or sale of a practice, there are two principal issues that come forward. One is governance and the other is compensation, (i.e., power and money). When there has been a takeover, a sale or merger of a practice, the issues have to do with cash put in or monies paid out to the physician selling and how the payout will be funded. The last principal issue that comes forth has to do with shared responsibility for call after hours, patient care, and practice management. The physicians in the group will need to determine how call responsibility, day-to-day patient care, and practice management issues will be shared, and whether any credit will be given for time spent on practice management and marketing issues in determining productivity and compensation.

When selling a practice, keep in mind that there are few hard assets available. An independent appraisal needs to be done to establish the valuation for real estate, furniture, and fixtures. Keep in mind that the principal assets of the practice really are the reputation, the goodwill, and the patient base of the individual physicians.

Under the current environment, medical records have little value, since there is a lower level of assurance that patients will stay with the succeeding practice and the high degree of risk that patients will leave the practice and follow the direction of their managed care contracts. Primary care practices have more value because of their attractiveness to managed care plans. When it comes to selling a practice, as with any business, the value is driven by the needs of the buyer. A hospital looking to buy a practice to build its primary care network is going to be paying more than another physician practice would. A hospital or managed care organization might be willing to spend heavily to acquire a practice to meet its market share and other business needs.

In selling a practice, a clearly defined sales contract needs to be drawn up. Most importantly, there needs to be a clear definition of what is being purchased:

- Assets.
- Medical records.
- Accounts receivable.
- Liabilities.
- Real estate.
- Leases (can these be assumed?).
- Name of the practice.

A noncompete clause also will have considerable value to a physician, and in some valuation methodologies will constitute the bulk of the purchase price. A noncompete clause typically will be one to two years in length and will stipulate a geographic range of a common market area, forbidding the physician from opening a new practice within the period covered by the agreement.

In the event of the sale of a practice that is still active, an employment contract typically will come along with the sale, guaranteeing the physician's income, benefits, and perhaps bonuses for a period of three to five years after the sale.

The valuation of a professional practice must be within the range of the fair market value (FMV), based upon an arm's length negotiation process. As noted earlier, independent appraisals are necessary in order to establish the value of any assets.

The Department of Health and Human Services, through the Office of the Inspector General (OIG), is concerned about using the sale price of a practice as a guise for making a payment to induce the continuation of referrals. It should be noted that, even if a physician is an employee of a practice owned by a hospital, she cannot be compelled to continue to refer to that organization. The areas the OIG will be concentrating on include the valuation of goodwill, the value of ongoing business, the value of noncompete covenants, and exclusive dealing in the value of patient lists and records.

As with any other merger or sale, the acquisition sale of a physician practice requires a significant amount of due diligence by the buyer. Due diligence is the process of gathering information to better understand, anticipate, and resolve issues and problems. In this stage of the due diligence process, the buyer will be developing forecasts of the business and financial performance of the operation. Goals of the process include understanding the operations and culture in order to effectuate the merger and consolidations. You will want to identify legal and regulatory compliance liabilities and issues and identify and understand clinical practice issues, including utilization practice patterns, and the like. The latter is important to ensure that the practice being acquired or merged with is consistent with your own organization and that its professional practices are of an ethical and professional nature and will not run you afoul of regulatory agencies later on.

As part of the due diligence process, you will include:

- Articles of incorporation and shareholders' agreements.
- Financial statements (at least three years' worth).
- Tax returns and tax matters at issue for the last three years.
- Obligations (such as leases and mortgages; liens; contracts, including employment, purchasing, and union contracts; employee benefits; and a listing of all employees and their wage rates, hours, and benefits).
- Licenses, permits, and other filings.
- All insurance policies in effect.
- Litigation known or anticipated.
- All properties held, both real estate and personal.

- All procedure and admission volumes.
- An audit or sample of the patient charts.

PLAYERS IN AN INTEGRATED SYSTEM

As discussed above, the nirvana of the organization of health care delivery services today is the so-called integrated delivery system (IDS) network. The five components of this integrated system are as follows:

- Hospitals.
- Physicians.
- Payer.
- Management company.
- Alternative sites and other nonphysician providers.

Let's take these one by one.

Hospitals

Hospitals need a strong alliance with physicians and payers in order to direct the patient flow. Neither hospitals nor payers admit or treat patients. Both parties need the primary care and specialty physicians in order to have any business.

Physicians

Physicians need access to capital in order to expand the services provided. Physicians, as noted above, do not have access to the equity markets but instead are dependent upon the ability to generate working capital internally or from additional cash investments from the partner physicians.

Payers

The payers bring the expertise in financing and administrating health benefits into the integrated network. Some hospitals are beginning to integrate with payers. For example, some hospitals own their own HMOs. At the time of this writing, Columbia/HCA is pursuing the acquisition of the Blue Cross/Blue Shield Plan of Ohio.

The Management Company

Management services organizations (MSOs) provide management services on a contract basis to physician groups. They can bring to the table an access to capital and economies of scale by serving multiple locations. In a typical setting, the management company will employ all of the office staff and support staff and own all the assets, including all leases for the facilities as well as diagnostic equipment. In the IDS model, the MSO would operate the physician practices that are owned or managed by the IDS organization or one of its components.

Alternative Site and Other Nonphysician Providers

These providers round out the comprehensive scope of services required in order to deliver the benefit package offered by the payers. The emphasis in health care delivery is to push the site of delivery down to the cheapest level. These alternative site providers include everything from home healthcare agencies and freestanding birthing centers to ambulatory surgery centers, freestanding imaging centers, labs, freestanding MRI centers, and rehab centers. Heretofore, investment dollars have flowed as the companies have been formed to combine the cottage industry of very small providers and to leverage the economies of scale into lower costs and higher profits.

Most commonly, physician practices looking at integration face four potential suiters:

- Physician–hospital organizations (PHOs).
- Management services organizations (MSOs) also known as physician practice management companies (PPMCs).
- Sale to a hospital.
- Acquisition by or merger with another practice.

Let's look at each of these suiters:

Physician–Hospital Organizations (PHO)

PHOs entail a low level of risk for all parties. Principally, they have been designed as a vehicle for managed care contracting, although they have in some instances been expanding and diversifying their activities. Much more so than the MeSH organizations of the 1980s, PHOs do align the interests of the hospitals and physicians in the goal of garnering a flow of patients directed by managed care organizations (MCOs). In order to succeed, PHOs must develop the utilization review and quality assurance functions, because, fundamentally, the key to the success of the MCO is the ability to control utilization. More advanced, mature PHOs have begun to provide billing services, management information services (MIS), and some management or MSO functions.

The structure of a PHO typically is one in which the board of directors contains equal representation from the hospital and the participating physicians. The capitalization to get these corporations underway must come from both parties. Very importantly, the return on investment must be based upon the financial performance of the PHO. If reimbursement is based on other criteria, particularly if it is geared toward rewarding physicians for referrals, whether explicitly or de facto, this would be considered a fraud and abuse matter and a kickback. That is the kind of activity that sank a number of imaging centers, ambulatory surgery centers, and other investment deals derived during the 1980s. Even though a PHO can entail a partnership between a not-for-profit, tax-exempt hospital and for-profit, tax paying physicians, the Internal Revenue Service (IRS) has ruled in some instances that such PHO arrangements can be organized as a not-for-profit, tax-exempt corporation. Again, the locality may still attempt to derive tax revenues regardless of the IRS ruling.

A PHO is an active management company and must include a committee structure, including finance, contracting, and, very importantly, medical advisory functions.

Successful PHOs are characterized by a number of characteristics, including:

1. Strong governance in management. The organization must be able to act decisively between its management staff and the board. All decisions cannot be subject to review by the entire membership.

2. Adequate capitalization (which is true with any business).
3. Strong physician support and leadership, particularly from the primary care physicians. This is all critical to maintain the support of the medical staff for the PHO so that its actions to control utilization will be acceptable to the membership.
4. Strong management information and utilization management systems. These are the heart of a successful contracting relationship with an MCO.
5. The ability to provide some selectivity of physicians to support the utilization management targets.

When you sign with a PHO, make sure that it is guaranteed that your practice will be provided with a copy of all contracts entered into promptly. There have been, and continues to be, a number of instances where PHOs and IPAs have not delivered copies of contracts to their members, yet the members were expected to accept patients and bill for services. In some cases, the members have not even been notified as to the existence of the contract. Practice staffs must sometimes be aggressive in obtaining the contracts and necessary information from the PHO and IPA staff.

Joining the PHO of the hospital, or hospitals, which are used by the practice often intuitively makes sense. As the payer community moves towards global types of risk contracts, the provider panels for a particular MCO are increasingly likely to come from a PHO type organization. Much as with the decision to sign on with a MCO, there usually is little risk to a practice to joining, and there is usually an "escape" i.e., a means to withdraw.

Management Services Organizations (MSO)

There are a variety of models of management service organizations (MSOs). Historically, we have been most familiar with the bookkeeping service, which handles the accounts payable for a practice and perhaps handles payroll. The MSO provides more sophisticated management services. Beyond basic bookkeeping, it provides better financial management and reporting services and the billing and collection service, again, something which we are familiar with from outside billing services. The MSO may be involved in the management of the office, including the employment of all the nonprofessional staff, the leasing of equipment and office space, and the purchasing function. Lastly, and what is often essential to MSO contracting, is the task of soliciting and developing networks and contracting with managed care organizations.

There are a number of MSO models, including:

- Freestanding, for-profit organizations, such as the large publicly-traded companies of Phycor and MedPartners.
- Hospital-affiliated MSOs, which have been acquiring more practices.
- Physician-affiliated MSOs, where one practice may provide management services to a multitude of practices.
- Joint ventures between hospitals and physicians, such as the PHO organization.
- Payer owned or affiliated organizations.

MSOs are not providers or suppliers of professional services and, as such, they simply act as agents on behalf of the physician practice. If there is a transfer of assets when the MSO essentially acquires the practice, the assets must be valued at fair market value and may only include the assets that a nonprofessional can own. The fee structure cannot be such that it will be construed as a kickback or an inducement to referrals. Insurers must be particularly cognizant of that. The antireferral and fraud and abuse laws come very much into play with an MSO.

When it comes to setting up a contract with an MSO, the critical part of the contract, as with any contract, is what the parties are agreeing to do. In this instance, what scope of services will the MSO be responsible for providing? It can be as simple as entailing only certain financial reporting or billing services and as complex as including ownership and responsibility for everything except the direct provision of professional medical care.

The contract should include a term and a termination point. Very often, these contracts have a very long term, anywhere from 5 to 40 years in length.

Fees can be determined in a number of ways, but it must be defined how these fees will be determined. For example, it could be a percentage of revenue or collections. There may be penalties for accounts that age too long as an incentive for the MSO to collect.

Also, the contract must specify the level of responsibility that the MSO will have in controlling expenses in order to ensure sufficient profits for the physician partners.

There should be a section in the contract dealing with the confidentiality of patient records, applicable to the manager and the MSO staff. The contract needs to spell out clearly the obligations of the physicians to support the MSO's information needs and reports and comply with procedures and legal requirements.

Since the MSO is acting in the name of the physicians, the physicians need to retain the right to approve its forms and letters and ensure the ethical behavior of the MSO and its staff.

Finally, there should be sufficient liability insurance taken by the MSO to indemnify the physicians for any actions the MSO takes that may reflect and put the physicians at risk.

The Hospital

Hospitals have gone on a buying binge for physician practices, particularly primary care practices, as a means of protecting patient referrals and to build the component pieces to contract with MCOs on a global fee basis. As the number of acquired practices grow, hospitals often will establish a division within the hospital, a MSO company, or turn over to a PHO the management of the practices. Hospitals, particularly ones that are new to practice acquisition, are not inherently adept at managing practices. Hospitals are organized around a larger bureaucracy than private practice physicians are used to. Physicians who sell their practice to a hospital will find that decision making is slower and sometimes more conservative.

The upside for a hospital as a suitor is that it is often a known quantity and its interests are usually centered on the local community. Physicians often will carry influence in hospital decision making and have access to senior management. For both parties (the hospital and the practice) the goal is a flow of patients, their timely and effective treatment and care, and discharge back to the community. A great many physicians have chosen this route.

Merger with another practice

Practices that choose to be autonomous can still grow and thrive, but they should be prepared to look at either growing through acquisition, or to be acquired themselves. Whether the acquirer, the acquired, or a merger of equals, bringing together professional practices is a difficult undertaking. Medical practices have the added dimension that the individual professionals are often dependent upon one another to provide the services to the practice's patients. The heart of a successful group practice is that the physicians come together as a group, covering for each other, collaborating on quality assurance activities, and sharing the leadership responsibilities in the health care and business community.

A larger practice, however, does require more management discipline and staff. Physicians will be ceding some of their authority and responsibility to professional managers who will have a closer handle on the day-to-day operation of the practice. For physicians considering a growth strategy, these dimensions need to be understood and accepted in order to this strategy to work. The physician owners also must collaborate and consult with others in the management decisions of the practice. The informality and closeness of a smaller organization is lost. Many are comfortable with these changes, others may not be. Those in the latter group must recognize this and either change, or pursue other strategies.

Appendix D is a Medical Practice Business Plan Workbook, designed as a step-by-step process to help a practice develop a business plan. A business plan, in its essence, is a process of learning about the business and the world around it, asking questions, probing for answers, identifying the options, making decisions, and then, most importantly, making the action plan—the business plan—come to life.

Throughout this book, I've suggested dozens of pieces of information to gather about your practice. In the workbook, I've tried to pull these together into a orderly process to build a "portrait" of the practice: its people, its customers, its markets, and an action plan to implement. One theme that runs through the workbook is viewing the practice in terms of the four critical resources:

- Human: the people and their skills.
- Physical: the facilities necessary for the organization to operate.
- Financial: financial resources, including cash available and debt capacity.

- Information and technology: hardware and software components of information systems; technological equipment and processes.

Each of these resources is assessed in the course of completing the workbook in terms of current capabilities and future needs.

In the end, a business plan comes down to management decisions. The learning process of the plan—the gathering of data from various sources—gives management a foundation for decision making. This is also a time to make, revise, or establish procedures within the practice to develop, report, and analyze this data on an ongoing basis. Information is power, it is said, and information is also comfort that "things are under control."

9

CHAPTER

Marketing the Practice

What is marketing? Marketing is a social and managerial process by which individuals and groups obtain what they need and want through creating an exchange in products and values with others.[1]

All organizations market in some manner or form. The standard definition of marketing includes the "four Ps:" product, price, place, promotion. Marketing is much more than advertising. In fact, advertising is only a very small part of what marketing is.

Marketing answers the following questions:

- Who are you?
- What do you do?
- Where can I find you?
- When can I meet you?
- When can you help me?
- How much will it cost?
- How can you help me?
- Why should I choose you?

There is a classic ad from McGraw-Hill magazines showing an angry old man with a scowl on his face, sitting in his chair with

[1] See Philip Kotler and Gary Armstrong, *Principles in Marketing*, 5th ed. (Englewood Cliffs, NJ: Prentice-Hall, 1991) for a more detailed discussion of marketing.

his cane, asking a series of similar questions. Marketing is a means of communicating what an organization can offer in terms of services and products to meet the needs and wants of an individual.

Marketing professional services is very different from the more traditional product marketing that we are familiar with for packaged goods such as cereal, soap powder, and the like. The product being offered by a professional service is not a physical object but in fact the skill, experience, judgment, and relationship of the professional himself. Professional services are relationship driven so that marketing is in fact inherent in any successful professional practice. In the traditional model, a new physician would start out by hanging around the emergency room looking to pick up the cases of those patients without a regular physician. In doing so, he also became known to the rest of the medical staff, who might then begin to refer patients to this new physician, particularly if they themselves were booked or unavailable. Some specialties have developed an ethos of being more aggressive in their marketing, particularly ophthalmology, where the patient uses more discretion in selecting the service or choosing to pursue a service. More aggressive marketing is also particularly true for radial keratotomy (RK) surgery, psychiatry, substance abuse treatment, and dentistry.

Central to the concept of marketing are two things: needs and wants. Needs are a state of felt deprivation regarding some human need, such as the physical need for food, shelter, and clothing; the social need for belonging and affection; and the individual need for knowledge and self-expression. Wants, on the other hand, are the form taken by needs as shaped by the culture and a person's individual personality. There can be more than one satisfier of a particular need. The consumer attempting to get the most satisfaction for the money and purchasing power he has available is creating demand. A product is anything that can be offered to a market that might satisfy a need or want. A product choice set is all those products that might satisfy a need or want.

Let's look at the four Ps: product, price, place, and promotion. Later, we'll return to the four Ps and discuss them from a marketing perspective.

1. Product is what the organization does—the services or goods it produces and offers to the market for consumption. The product of a medical practice is the entire scope of the interaction between the physician, the practice, and the patient: the services offered, how it is offered, and where it is offered. Medical practices, by their nature, provide their product in a number of locations and rely upon other organizations to support and otherwise provide part of the services that make up the "product" of medical care. For the practice, the components of the product include: extended office hours, additional offices, in-house radiology and lab, affiliated hospitals, and the use of midwives and midlevel practitioners. The practice also depends upon independent clinical laboratories, outside imaging centers, hospitals, and other specialists to provide some of the services that all come together in what the patient—the customer—perceives as the "product."

2. Price. Price is reflected as both the cost and the value. Most products have one price for all buyers but, in health care, there may be different prices for different buyers. The pricing decision, therefore, is tied to the distribution channel, that is, whether a patient is coming in on her own as opposed to being referred and directed by a managed care organization.

A price is determined based upon the cost plus a fair rate of return. There may be multiple factors that affect pricing decisions, including quantity, the buyer's perceived value, economic conditions, competition, and other marketing considerations. Physician services often have been priced without a solid foundation or rational analysis. To the degree, it has been a matter of what the market will bear; however, it often has no relationship to what in fact the market does bear. Where insurance coverage pays for services, the actual payment received by the physician may vary considerably from the posted charge or price. As a result, the real price can be different and lower than the posted charge.

3. Place (distribution). The concepts of place and distribution concern how to connect the buyer with the product. Historically, in health care physician services have been determined directly by the consumer with the payer acting as simply the payment source providing the cash. In the new reality of health care, however, the payer is interjected in this process and becomes a middleman or wholesaler, receiving groups of patients from employers and "selling" these groups to physicians and other providers in bulk.

Physicians are distributors for hospitals and hospital services. The only person who can make a decision to admit a patient to a hospital (which then generates the "sale" of hospital services) is a physician.

The last ones in the food chain are the primary care physicians, who are the distributors for the specialists' services. Again, particularly in managed care arrangements, the gatekeeper primary care physician determines from which specialist the services will be purchased.

Places of service and distribution channels include offices; hospitals; phone, fax, and wireless forms of communication; group practices; alternative site facilities, such as mobile mammography, mobile nuclear imaging, and other kinds of mobile imaging services; and telemedicine.

4. Promotion. Promotion is any means of communication with customers and suppliers about your organization, its products, services, what it stands for, its pricing, and its competitive qualities. Means of promotion include advertising, public relations (which includes special events, media interviews, and educational events), personal selling, promotions (such as coupons), and special pricing. An example of special pricing would be a special, low fee charged for a mammogram and physical exam during the National Cancer Society's Breast Cancer Awareness Day.

THE PROMOTIONAL MIX

The promotional mix is the combination of efforts in these different areas which together achieve the goals for promotion of the product, service, or organization. The marketing mix reflects the various degrees of activities and investments in product, price, place, and promotion that are the core of an organization and what it does.

The key questions facing the organization, then, in making marketing happen include:

- Who are my customers?
- What makes them different and what makes them alike?
- How will I communicate with them?
- What do I want to tell them?
- What are my goals in marketing?

That's the focus. The key question is: What are my goals? As with most activities within an organization, the fundamental, underlying question is: What am I trying to achieve? It is important to understand that marketing is very much a process—a process of learning, planning, and doing.

UNDERSTANDING THE MARKETPLACE

The first step in marketing and marketing planning involves pulling together the data available to the organization. In professional services such as health care, demographic information is critically important in understanding the marketplace and making projections for future demand. Demographic data are available in a number of forms, most commonly from a number of demographic service bureaus around the country, including CACI, National Decision Systems, Dun & Bradstreet, and others. All demographic data are fundamentally based upon the U.S. Census, which is conducted every 10 years. The census data are based upon census tracks, which are small areas of land and population. The census bureau supplements the census with specialized surveys that are ongoing throughout the decade in between census publications. The demographic service bureaus take those data, update them and make estimates in different geographic boundaries, most commonly using zip codes. The bureaus use information such as driver's license data, home construction and moving information, and birth and death rates in order to make these estimates. They typically will give you current estimated data as well as five-year projected data. Their data also can be mapped and presented based on any geographic coordinate point. However, the most commonly used boundaries are political boundaries or zip codes, as well as a radius from a given geographic point, say the intersection of two roads. This gives you potential demographic information by age group for a potential market service area. It is important to note that this information is an estimate and that there are flaws, even in the U.S. Census. The smaller the population base of a given area, the more likely and the more significant will be a variance or error. In inner city areas, the U.S. Census reportedly has numerous problems in undercounting, particularly in poor and immigrant communities. Regardless, the census information has a fairly good foundation in fact and, as they say, it is close enough for government work.

From your perspective as a physician practice, you are looking to map out your service area. Using the internal database in your computer system, you can look at the number of patients whose residences are in a given service area. This will tell you the number of patients per thousand population in your practice. Then, you can compare this with the total patients per thousand population, which often can be estimated using data from your professional society. From this information, you now can estimate your market share for a given geographic area. The demographics should be done based upon the typical age bands: 0–17, 18–44, 45–64, 65–74, and 75 plus. Depending upon your specialty, you may find your patients fall into different age brackets. For example, pediatricians obviously have a larger patient base in the under 18 group; an obstetrician has a higher percentage of 18 to 44-year-old females; a cardiologist has more patients in the 45 and over group; and so on. At age 65 and over, utilization begins to climb significantly. In the 75 and over population, both male and female, there is a geometric increase in utilization of physician and other diagnostic testing services.

Your utilization by CPT code also should be compiled at this time. Using your computer system, you should be able to generate the utilization by CPT code for each zip code. While it makes intuitive sense that the distribution among CPT codes should be fairly consistent from zip code to zip code area, if you cover a wide geographic area or multiple hospitals, you may find that emergency type situations are clustered in zip codes closest to the hospital where you are principally affiliated or where you do most of your work. If there are variances, you may find that, if you are a specialist, some of your specialty work is being done by primary care physicians or competing specialists in other geographic areas more distant from your practice office. Regardless, this information is important and fairly easy to extract, and it is simply one of the base points you will need to check as you proceed through your planning and marketing process.

In this age of managed care, with its emphasis on patient satisfaction and quality of care, market research activities may be helpful in providing some basis for your decisions and analysis.

Market research has a scientific basis but there is much subjective measurement that goes on. Market research is used to test concepts, measure success, and analyze markets and consumers. The tools used in market research include:

- Surveys, both written and by telephone.
- Focus groups.
- Personal interviews.
- Test marketing.

Let's look at some of these tools in some depth.

Surveys

Surveys have varying degrees of scientific basis and statistical veracity, depending upon how they are conducted. It is important to understand that in all market research, measurement is an interpretation and is not as precise as we would find in clinical and other diagnostic testing situations. Often, a large degree of subjective measurement and decision making go into the analysis; hence, it is more the art of marketing rather than the science of marketing. The same could hold true, of course, in medical practice where there is still a large degree of judgment based upon the clinical information being presented.

Survey forms come in two kinds: one that is returned by mail, and one that is completed on-site. Anonymous surveys tend to have better response rates and provide better information. However, surveys filled out on-site (when a patient is in the office, for example), tend to get a high return rate. Surveys mailed to people at random can hope for a 1 to 2 percent return. The idea behind all surveys is that they are done at random; in other words, there is some randomness in the selection of who fills them out. Telephone surveys are another way to conduct a survey; however, in the medical arena, having nonpractice employees make the calls brings into question the degree of confidentiality you have maintained. I once was involved in conducting a survey for a hospital, in which it provided a random list of former patients and their telephone numbers. When the market research firm went to make the calls, it began by asking for a specific individual's name. The problem was twofold: (1) it was asking for an individual; and

(2) it was hitting a large number of unlisted numbers. The research firm had to change the survey and simply ask for someone who might have been a patient in a hospital.

Important features to consider in selecting a telephone survey firm include: (1) the degree of confidentiality; and (2) whether the firm will first test your survey using a small group of perhaps 10 to 15 people. There invariably will be kinks in your survey (i.e., a question that seems perfectly clear to you, the author of the survey, may be interpreted quite differently by the person asking and the person answering the question). This test allows you to then revise the questionnaire to be more precise.

Focus groups

Focus groups are a gathering of a small group (about a dozen) of customers for the purposes of discussing a product, company, or issue. Their is considerable debate as to the value of the information that comes out of focus groups, for it is based on discussion and impression rather than a more research based methodology. Focus groups work by gathering a group, often chosen from a random sample, together into a room. A facilitator leads the discussion, trying to prevent any one person or any one opinion from dominating or steering the discussion. Focus groups are usually put together and lead by a market research firm. The discussion is recorded, usually on videotape, and the client's representatives may watch through a one way mirror.

Focus groups are useful for probing into a limited number of topics, such as certain areas which have a high negative finding in a patient satisfaction survey. For new or expanding services, it can lend some insight into what will or will not be of interest to patient, and more importantly, the format allows a good facilitator to probe the why behind the questions and opinions.

Personal interviews

Personal interviews are best used when the opinions of specific individuals are desired, or the depth and detail of the information and opinion sought will take a longer time to elicit. When developing a business plan for a medical practice, personal interviews might be done with other specialists, senior hospital management and leading business and human resources executives in the community.

Demographic and Market Information

There are a number of pieces of demographic and market information that are important to gather as part of this stage of your marketing and planning process. In addition to straight demographic data for market share, demographic data also present societal trends that may have an impact. Looking at trends over time will tell you whether you have a population that is aging, both as a percentage of the total population, as well as in hard numbers. For example, a physician may choose to specialize in serving the elderly. In a very fast growing market, the physician may find that, on a percentage basis, the percentage of elderly is flat or declining but, in real numbers, the market is growing. So even though the percentage basis and the total market share of elderly are declining, there is sufficient growth in hard numbers that it still could be a very attractive opportunity for this physician.

Historical data (going back at least three years as to volumes of utilization and estimated market share) are the next to gather. Other trends in society in the market area include household formations and specific geographic areas of growth (for example, is the northern part of the city growing while the southern part of the city is losing population?).

Finally, competitor intelligence, meaning information as to the actions of potential and current competitors, always should be watched. News clippings are an easy way to watch your competitors' actions. Classified ads also will give you some indication as to new hirings, rapid turnover, and perhaps new services. As an example, when I was in Pittsburgh a competing hospital began to advertise for waitresses for a special unit in its hospital. Although no public announcement had been made, it obviously was opening up a "gold coast" unit similar to what we had been planning.

SEGMENTATION AND POSITIONING

There are two concepts in marketing that are important to understand: segmentation and positioning. Segmentation is classifying customers into groups with different needs, characteristics, and/or behavior. A market segment is a group of customers who responds in a similar way to a given set of marketing stimuli (marketing stimuli being advertising, coupons, educational programs, or other kinds of promotional activities). A market segment, therefore, is a grouping of people with common needs, wants, and characteristics, such as demographics, personality traits, incomes, lifestyles, and geographic location.

Positioning is the targeting of your product or service to a particular market segment or segments. Positioning, in a nutshell, is perception. The classic comment on positioning was made by Charles Revson, the founder of the Revlon cosmetic company. Revlon, as you are no doubt aware, produces dozens of types of cosmetics and perfumes. When asked about the products, Mr. Revson answered, "What I sell is hope." Although the basic ingredients in many perfumes are fairly common, the cost of ingredients and manufacturing are but a very small part of the sales price of the product. Packaging, the use of white-coated sales clerks, and luxurious ads all position the product in the mind of the consumer and that imply, by using it, a glamorous lifestyle will be her's.

Hospitals have tried to do the same thing and position themselves as high-tech hospitals with the latest equipment and the most advanced medical staff. Albert Einstein Medical Center in Philadelphia goes so far as to use as its tag line, "Genius in health care," next to the drawing of its namesake, Albert Einstein.

Now let's discuss the four Ps in more detail:

Marketing: The Product

Professional services such as medical practices are *personal* services; that is, you, the professional, are the product. The professional is the product in the sense of his training, experience, skill, ability to relate to people, and responsiveness to the demands and requests of his patients. Clients and patients rely upon the professional for advice, counsel, and direct service, a laying on of the hands in treatment. What we have seen in this country over the past few years is the commoditization of professional services, that is, in the minds of many consumers, there is little difference between professional A and professional B, that is, between physician A and physician B. For professionals, it is very difficult to demonstrate a real difference in quality of service, particularly when it comes to medical care. Other than the services available at academic centers, hospitals and physicians are hard-pressed to differentiate why they are better than the other guy. As we discuss marketing in these pages, please remember that there are many components that go into making someone a better physician. Very often, a better match between the physician and the patient will lead to better care, better outcomes and higher patient satisfaction—more so than a pure demonstration of qualitative superiority of one physician over another, clinical care rendered, and/or the judgments made. Again, the professional service is a personal relationship.

Other aspects that comprise the product include everything surrounding the service. One is the appearance and accessibility of your office. As mentioned elsewhere in this book, I once walked into an interview for a new practice being formed and found the waiting room decorated with those posters that show the minimum wage law, worker's compensation rights, and the like. I never did get to ask why these posters were in the reception room and, had I been offered the position, my first act would have been to take them down! Office cleanliness and tidiness are all aspects of the product. A plastic surgeon who positions himself as the "plastic surgeon of the stars" is going to invest in more glamorous and glitzy surroundings than will a primary care physician serving a middle class population. A Pittsburgh hospital that serves women exclusively set up a series of outpatient mammography centers. In these centers, the setting was both feminine and upscale. Walls were decorated with nice wallpaper, the waiting area offered comfortable, noninstitutional chairs, and coffee and tea were served on real china, as opposed to the typical paper or styrofoam cup or drug company mug. This is perhaps best summarized by Donald Burr, president of People's Express Airline, the low cost startup from the 1980s. He said, "Coffee stains on the flip down trays mean bad maintenance on the airplanes."

Other aspects of the product are very much centered around your staff, for it has more interaction than anyone else. A comment that someone made to me years ago about hospital care was that, "Patients are admitted to hospitals for nursing care, not medical care."

Other aspects include attentiveness to patients, responsiveness to calls or requests for assistance, and the timeliness of the schedule. Patients are the lifeblood of a practice. You have heard this. This must be an integral part of how your practice operates and how you and your staff treat your patients. Phone calls and requests for assistance by patients, be it filling out insurance forms, obtaining copies of their records, or receiving simple advice are all part of the treatment and care process. Physicians are trained to believe in the personal relationship between themselves and their patients. What is discussed in these pages is very much a part of that relationship and is what bonds the physician and the patient together. I can not emphasize enough the importance of keeping to the schedule and using one that is tuned to balancing the needs of the practice as well as the patient. If your practice develops a reputation for running late all the time, patients will start coming late as a rule, which will further exacerbate the problem. If you are late, apologize. If you are constantly late, change your scheduling.

Like it or not, your participation in health plans, including managed care organizations and the acceptance of Medicare assignments is a part of the product. Patients who have a managed care plan as their health plan cannot and will not go to you. On the contrary, they will drop you if forced to obtain the benefits of the plan. Medicare assignment is simply an indication of your willingness to stay with patients throughout their lifetime.

The last aspect of the product concerns hospital privileges. Hospitals have become competitive over the years in marketing directly to patients, trying to influence them to select their hospital of choice rather than simply rely on their physician's recommendation. Managed care plans, because of their contracting networks, have preselected hospitals where all their patients will go. As a result, your ability to join the medical staffs of hospitals where you will be directed to send patients becomes another component of your product and service.

Historically, maternity patients were the only ones who would focus on selecting a hospital as part of their process of selecting an obstetrician. As patients have become more sophisticated, the availability of certain hospitals, particularly university hospitals for tertiary care, factors more often into the physician selection equation.

Marketing: The Price

Pricing is in fact an issue for many patients. The charge often made is that one of the reasons why health care costs have increased so dramatically in this country is that patients pay for nothing—that, in fact, insurance pays for most health care expenses. The reality of course is far different, that there are a large number of small costs that do accrue to patients.

Principal among these is prescription drugs. Many indemnity plans do not cover the cost of prescription drugs or, if they do, they fall under the same pattern of coverage as all general medical care; after a deductible, the company will pay 80 percent of usual and customary reimbursement (UCR). Managed care plans typically will provide prescription drug coverage under two or three groupings: generic, preferred, and nonpreferred. The generic drug class is as it implies; it includes those drugs that are available in generic form. The preferred drug class is often offered when the health plan, or more likely a prescription benefit manager, has access to significantly discounted pricing. The third class, nonpreferred, includes drugs that are name brand, for which significant savings have not been able to be negotiated. In addition, for the preferred class, the drug may be cheaper than the nonpreferred drug, and the plan may have been able to negotiate a better discount by guaranteeing greater volumes.

Physicians should review their most commonly prescribed drugs with the plans so that at least they are aware under which class these drugs fall. The physician may find that he is comfortable writing a preferred or even generic class prescription in many instances. If he needs to write a prescription for a nonpreferred drug as opposed to a generic drug, he may be questioned by the health plan from time to time or more likely by his patients. Being prepared with a clinical basis for these decisions at least supports the choice.

Prescription drug plans are often "carved out" and managed by prescription benefit managers. These are companies that specialize in managing, as the name implies, the prescription drug benefit piece of the health plan. These companies are one of the many companies that have captured a piece of the health care continuum and focused on economies of scale and volume buying in order to produce maximum benefits for customers and maximum profits for shareholders. Medco Containment is one of the largest and most well known partially because it was acquired by Merck Pharmaceutical a few years ago. These companies often maintain mail order prescription houses to fill long-term chronic medication needs. The mail order option may or may not be part of the health plan, since it usually provides 30-day-plus prescriptions.

Other patient issues concern pricing the required copayments, determining any deductibles, and finally premium sharing. As a general rule, managed care plans significantly reduce the out-of-pocket expenses to a healthy patient and only in the event of an illness do the deductibles come into play. This is consistent with the underpinnings of insurance generally, where you only pay out-of-pocket when you have had a loss. This is contrary to how indemnity plans work; in these plans, you begin paying on the first dollar, and all health care is in effect a medical loss.

All in all, the principal buyers of health care services are the health care plans and the employers. As has been discussed earlier in this book, the reason why managed care plans have grown so dramatically is simply because of the big push by employers to crank down their health care costs. And guess what? They have been successful.

Marketing: The Place

The push to reduce healthcare costs by lowering utilization is backed by the push of moving healthcare services down to the least expensive setting. Although in most communities the hospital still remains the center of the healthcare system (due to its sheer size and resources, both physical and in terms of people skills), there are a variety of alternative sites that have become the focus of more and more healthcare services. From a physician's perspective, in order to market herself successfully, she needs to be able to utilize the various levels of sites available. By participating in health plans, a physician ensures the greater coverage of possible payers for employers and patients. Since the health plan now enters into the healthcare decision-making process, the plan determines what universe of providers will be providing services.

The key issue then is your membership on the necessary hospital staffs. While as a general rule you want to keep your hospital staff memberships to a minimum, you may need to make arrangements to cover more than one hospital in order to cover the needs of the health plan and your patients. This, of course, is where the advantages of a group practice come into play, for physicians can split up principal responsibility for different hospitals.

Accessibility is another key issue in the place part of marketing. Whether you have only one office location or more than one location, your office should be readily accessible to patients. If your office is a specialist facility and you are the least bit difficult to find, one way to help matters is to provide your referring physicians with preprinted referral pads with your name and address and a map on the back with directions.

The appearance of your office is also very important. As indicated earlier, cleanliness and the presentation of a crisp, professional environment with some warmth to it are very important. The last thing you want today is a very sterile environment.

Medical offices typically work best when laid out as a square, minimizing the distances patients and staff have to walk to get from point A to point B. Very important, of course, is handicapped accessibility: hallways must be at least 36 inches wide at all points, including doorways. Your architect can lend assistance in the specifics and inform you of any local zoning requirements. The outside of the building needs to be ramped so that a wheelchair or someone who has difficulty walking can readily gain access to your building. Whether or not you own the building, this kind of access needs to be in place. Otherwise, do not select the building in the first place.

Pediatric practices or other practices that serve children should have a play area with good, safe toys. Bathrooms need to be equipped with changing areas and, again, need to be handicapped accessible. You may not necessarily need a public restroom for your patients in your office suite itself, but there should be one in close proximity.

One of the principal issues for managed care plans is the geographic availability of the provider network. Employers tend to be concentrated in a central city, but employees can live in any direction. In order to sell the insurance product, health plans must have a provider network that covers the areas where employees live. In some markets, people will travel as much as one to two hours each way to work, so the geographic circle of the provider network can get rather large. From the health plan's point of view, a provider who can address the geographic coverage challenge makes network building easier for the plan and helps the plan sell product. One of the strategic issues to consider is where and whether to add additional offices for the practice.

Marketing: Promotion

Promotion is the means by which you communicate with customers and other important publics. Promotion works by:

- Identifying your target audience, that is, the audience you are trying to reach.
- Determining what kind of response is sought. Are you looking for someone to make a buying decision? Are you looking for someone to make a phone call to request material?
- Choosing your message or what you are trying to convey to the audience.
- Selecting your media, for example, newspapers, radio, television, or mail.

In the next section of this chapter, let's focus our discussion on some of the practical aspects of promotion.

PRACTICAL ASPECTS OF PROMOTING THE PRACTICE

As noted above, promotion entails communication with customers and other important publics. Other important publics can include other physicians, hospitals and hospital staffs, the news media, health plans, and government agencies—in short, a whole host of people with whom you interact directly or indirectly in the course of managing a practice. More than likely, what you want to convey to this audience is that your practice is composed of skilled, compassionate, experienced physicians who provide first-rate quality medical care and have a human touch.

One of the most common ways of communicating is through a press release. Press releases are more than unpaid advertising. They are printed because they have some newsworthy value to the readers of the publication. The newspaper, for instance, will not publish every press release you send unless, in the editor's judgment, some significant portion of the readership will have some interest in reading it. This readership may be consumers who buy services from your practice as patients but also may include people who do business with your practice or potentially could do business with your practice. As a rule, press releases should be no more than one page in length. The opening paragraph is in the style of a newspaper article, answering the five key questions: Who, What, When, Where, and Why. You also should include a paragraph that describes a little bit about your organization and who you are. Press releases should definitely be double spaced with one-inch margins all around. The heading should include, in capital letters, "for immediate release." Most media outlets will not hold or embargo a press release unless you are a significant or very important organization. Press releases can be mailed, or they can usually be faxed. Tying up E-mail with a press release is probably not the best way to go. Several days after the release is sent, it is perfectly acceptable to follow up with a phone call to the editor to ensure it has been received and answer any questions. If the decision is made not to run it, it is best not to argue. Depending upon the size of your market, you may be able to ask for some advice as to how a press release could be structured to better fit the publication's needs. However, beyond that, there is not much you can do on a short term basis.

The Yellow Pages directory is the most common form of advertising for a practice. In the last several years, there has been a proliferation of "yellow pages." The Yellow Page name is considered generic, in that it does not belong exclusively to the local phone company. Newspapers, the R. R. Donnelley Printing Company, and others have come out with their own versions of local directories to compete with the local telephone company directory. This, of course, leads to a situation where you can easily double your expenditures in yellow pages with questionable value of return. You also may find that the geographic areas are being microsegmented. I have seen counties as small as 200,000 people where the phone company had three distinct yellow pages directories and expected clients to advertise in all three, effectively tripling our yellow pages expense. My response was, of course, to reduce the size of the ad and pull it from one directory.

Using the yellow pages in and of themselves as a source of new patients also is questionable, although the sales representatives will swear up and down that the yellow pages are the best means of advertising anything. The value of the yellow pages depends upon the location and the type of practice you have. Those which are discretionary and patient directed, such as plastic surgery and chiropractic practices, are more likely to be yellow pages driven than, say, the practices of an internist or neurosurgeon. One way of evaluating your yellow pages needs is to ask your patients how they found out about the practice and whether they have ever used the yellow pages to find a physician. You may find that people use the yellow pages to look up a phone number of a physician or to locate a physician within a particular practice that operates under another name.

Another means of communicating with your patients as they become patients of the practice is through what is called a "capability brochure." This brochure is a handout that can include the following:

- Biographies of the professional staff.
- The names and brief biographies of your support staff.
- The history and purpose of your organization.
- The services offered within your practice.
- The hours, office locations, and financial policies of the practice.

The capability brochure is an effective vehicle for you to tell current and prospective patients who you are, what you do, and a little about policies they need to be aware of, particularly financial policies.

A capability brochure can be made in several formats. A one piece booklet has the advantage of being one piece, and is neat and easy to carry and read. Its disadvantage is that changes cannot be made without reprinting the entire booklet. A folder based capability brochure/packet uses a folder with one or two inside pockets, allowing various printed materials to be inserted in the pockets. Folders come in several sizes, from $8^1/_2 \times 11$ inches on down to business envelope size. The inserts can be revised frequently, and the contents of each folder can be customized depending upon the intended uses and audience.

Desktop publishing software, which range from the simple to the complex, has dramatically cut the price of developing brochures. One technique for adding color to printed pieces is to print shells. "Shells" have no copy (written words) on them, only the color design and/or name of the organization is printed. A shell is much like letterhead. Since the cost of printing is in the setup, it can pay to print a large quantity of shells using color. Each insert is printed in one color only, and you can run smaller quantities, even using an in-house computer. For example, you may print 10,000 shells for use during a year. You use the shells, with the standardized design, to then print each of the inserts as needed. This minimizes your turnover and wastage and enables you to update your staff biographies and any policy changes as necessary.

There are a host of promotion opportunities available to a practice. Newspapers are one that most people think of very quickly but be careful, for this may not be the best outlet for your practice. The first question should be, "What am I trying to achieve?" Newspapers can document fairly well the population and the residence of their readership. However, they may cover an area of much wider geography than your potential patient base. In larger markets, the newspaper may publish regional editions, and you may have better success advertising in these. Some may only have regional inserts, that is, a special weekly section that is devoted to the geographic area, while the other sections of the paper are generic for the entire marketplace. You will want to target your area of interest and your particular customers as best as possible.

In newspaper advertising, you pay for your placement. ROP (run of paper) is the cheapest way to go in that the ad will be placed at the discretion of the editor. Preferred positioning, such as the upper right-hand corner of a right page, the back page of a section, or within a certain specialty section, (e.g., sports, television, and such) may entail a premium price. If you are trying to reach women, the style section is probably the best placement. If you are trying to reach business people, obviously the business section is your best bet. Men are best reached in the sports section. Science and health selections, when available, are best to reach educated consumers who take a stronger interest in their health care. My personal favorite is the weekly television section. My theory is that people tend to keep this section around for an entire week and refer to it frequently, thereby increasing the opportunities for an ad to be seen.

Certain national magazines also will have regional editions. Again, while you may place advertising in these sections, be aware that you are paying a very high price for a narrowly targeted audience.

Pennysaver or other similar weekly advertising newspapers are another way of reaching your potential patients. These papers, sometimes called "shoppers," contained pages of classified ads, usually from consumers selling used goods. Interestingly, these "shoppers" are looked at by many people.

Many larger markets also have local papers that contain news about very specific locations within the market as well as a lot of advertising. It is fairly easy to buy cheap advertising space or run an article under the guise of advertising. You may wish to explore this option as well.

Radio is one of the unsung heroes in many areas in terms of reaching potential consumers. Radio is very much a target medium, in that the format, be it music or talk, is generally targeted to a very specific demographic audience, which the radio stations will be pleased to tell you about. These stations also can tell you the peak and best listening times, which typically are the drive times. Drive times may run from about 6:00 AM to 10:00 AM and from 3:00 PM to 6:00 or 7:00 PM, depending upon the market and the degree of traffic. These timeframes have the highest listenership. Radio is also very locally focused. Even in the largest markets, there are local stations with a weaker signal that reach only the people they are trying to reach in their geographic area. For example, in New York City, WCBS–FM with 50,000 watts of power will reach upwards of 10,000,0000 people. If you were a practice based in the Queens section of New York City, buying advertising time on that station would be a huge waste unless you expected to be reaching patients from that entire market area. Since most health care is local, this is an unlikely event. A tertiary care hospital, however, may find such a station to be an excellent value.

In addition to advertising, opportunities with radio include interviews, expert interviews as a supplement to the news program, appearances on call-in shows, public service announcements, and public service programming.

There are a number of personal appearance outlets that you can use if you are someone who feels comfortable making presentations before an audience. In every town and every market, there are dozens of community groups that are always on the lookout for interesting speakers. These include Rotary Clubs, Kiwanis Clubs, sisterhoods, men's clubs, church and synagogue groups, YMCAs, JCCs, and such. Many enclosed shopping malls also sponsor walking clubs that may be interested in speakers who will spend five to ten minutes discussing a health related subject with the hardy corps of people out every morning walking in the mall. Hospitals often will fall over each other trying to be the sponsor of these walking clubs. Many communities also have health fairs and senior fairs, sometimes sponsored by shopping malls which offer opportunities to speak, to set up a booth for information and screening exams, as well as for sponsorship.

Sponsorships often are sought by community groups for everything from Little League teams and school sports teams to various festivals, plays, and school yearbooks. Many of these constitute what I call "must do" ads. These are goodwill types of arrangements that will cost you $50 to $100 each and allow you to make a small contribution to something in the community. On the one hand, you do need to take the position that you cannot place ads in every publication that is presented to you. By having a marketing strategy, you can always point to that in declining to make some of these contributions and selecting others. The question you must ask is, "Who are you trying to reach?"

For example, a pediatric practice might be making a wise investment in sponsoring a Little League team. A physician or a psychiatrist who specializes in treating adolescents might want to advertise and serve as a sponsor for high school yearbooks and plays. A specialty practice or a general practice serving principally adults, particularly in the 30 to 60 age group, may want to place most of its ads in community group plays or calendars and the like. The goal is to look for outlets for your name to appear in places that will be seen by the people you are trying to reach.

Unless you are a very large practice, television advertising, even on cable-only channels, is very expensive for the number of impressions you will reach for your potential return. Do note, however, that cable systems offer the opportunity to target a television spot very tightly. For example, a television signal will reach the entire market viewing area and cannot differentiate or have a regional edition. However, cable systems tend to be under a more narrowly defined geographic basis and will offer opportunities for advertising on some of the cable-only networks. A package I commonly see includes ESPN, CNN, Lifetime, USA, and TNT, all for one price.

Public television and community access television are other opportunities to consider. Community access has never enjoyed wide viewership. Even sponsoring your own program on such an outlet is one I would question as far as its value. Educational television is quite a different story. Although you cannot place a pure advertisement on these stations, you can be a sponsor or principal sponsor of certain programs, depending upon the audience you are trying to reach. If you are trying to reach the business community, the "Nightly Business Report" is one potentially good vehicle. If you are trying to reach children, "Sesame Street," "Barney," or "The Magic School Bus" may provide better opportunities for getting your message to the children as well as their parents, the decision makers.

Most professional services still very much rely upon a referral as the source of new business. All the promotional activities we are discussing in this section ultimately come down to a means of establishing name recognition and qualifications, in effect, setting the stage for the development of a personal relationship. Networking, therefore, is a highly effective tool that is often utilized with greatest success by consultants, accountants, attorneys, and the like. Involvement in any community organization, from Rotary Clubs and Kiwanis to your church or synagogue or civic action groups, brings you in contact with a wide number of people who are leaders in the community. These influencers also are then in a position to influence other people who may be looking for your services.

Someone once summed up to me the objective of networking as being, "Who you know and who you can get to know." Some of these organizations offer opportunities to sponsor an activity. As an example, the Chamber of Commerce in a number of locales offers businesses the opportunity to sponsor the monthly breakfast or lunch meeting. Typically, with this small fee, your name will be identified with every piece of promotional literature, you will have a few minutes to speak at the meeting, and you will be able to distribute materials at the table of every attendee. I have done this personally on several occasions, achieving what I believe to be good success through name recognition. In addition to a very brief speech, the practice left some literature at every table and also left a 32-ounce water bottle with the practice's logo emblazoned on it at every place setting. I was quite satisfied to see that almost all of the water bottles were taken home by the 200-plus attendees at the meeting. In using advertising specialties, you are competing with dozens upon dozens of giveaways every day. I believe in ad specialties but with the caveat to look for something that has some true utility and that people will keep. One of my favorites when I was at a large hospital in Pittsburgh was the use of 6-inch jar grippers, those thin pieces of rubber that are used to open a tightly-sealed jar. Everyone needs one but never has one. I gave away 12,000 to 15,000 jar grippers a year, many at an annual senior festival sponsored by the county area agency on aging. We received a number of phone calls from small community groups asking for donations of these jar grippers as giveaways at events they were holding. We were happy to comply under the theory that people would use these and keep them in a kitchen drawer, with the jar gripper emblazoned with our name and phone number. Mugs and note pads have their uses, and they are fairly cheap, but remember they are rather ubiquitous.

The United States has a long history of freedom of speech and self publishers publishing newsletters, monographs, flyers, and magazines. Recent technological developments have put the power of publishing into millions of more hands by introducing desktop computers and relatively inexpensive software, as well as offset printing. Newsletters have become a very popular form of communication and marketing by a wide variety of organizations from college alumni associations to Starbucks Coffee (which includes a newsletter with your coffee shipment), frequent flyer clubs, and professional service firms—in fact, just about anyone who has something to say. This author's experience has been that a good newsletter is looked at and read.

A newsletter offers a means of communicating timely information with your customers, which in this case include patients and physicians. In addition, the newsletter also can serve as a means of general promotion when sent to the media and other parties who influence medical decisions and medical information.

Certain specialists, such as primary care physicians and specialists who have an ongoing relationship with a patient, (such as psychiatry and cardiology) can be served by a good patient newsletter. A newsletter can be used to reinforce general lifestyle, health maintenance, and prevention advice, answer many of the common questions patients have, as well as reemphasize instructions given to many patients, such as using prescription medication, watching for side effects and danger signs in their particular illness, and the like.

For specialists who are very dependent upon referrals from other physicians, it makes sense to have a physician newsletter. In doing so, you must be very cognizant not to appear too sales-driven or flashy, for by and large this is somewhat anathema to physicians. Regardless, you can make it look nice and convey a message of expertise, knowledge, and professionalism.

Among the things that can be communicated in a specialist's newsletter include guidance for primary care physicians as to when a referral to a specialist may be appropriate, a decision that is confronted more frequently under a managed care environment. The tone of the newsletter cannot be preachy but it can be informational. The newsletter also can provide up-to-date information regarding new diagnosis and treatment techniques and possibilities, the latest studies, and case experience, both reported in the journals as well as experienced locally by the practice. The letter also can discuss community resources that primary care physicians can use and refer their patients to for information, education, and support.

In terms of general promotion, the message being conveyed is that the newsletter authors have an expertise in certain areas and can communicate effectively with a nonprofessional audience. It also may be the basis for a cover letter to a reporter suggesting where a piece of your newsletter might be incorporated in an article of their own. Obviously, the outcome here is that you would be interviewed and quoted in the newspaper article or media report. Newsletters are fairly inexpensive to produce. They do need to be printed on a good stock of paper. One of the ways to reduce your cost and still use one or two colors in addition to black type is by printing what are known as shells. As already mentioned above, shells are the first pass of the paper that have the color printed first. You can print a sufficient quantity of the shells with, say, your name, the newsletter title, and certain borders to last for one year. With each issue, you then typeset around the preprinted areas and print only in sufficient quantity for that issue. The rest of the shells are kept in stock. The reason this is done is that the cost in printing is all in the set-up, that is the stripping of the machines and the press, adding the color, and running the set-up. A printer needs to run a number of copies until the press gets going correctly. So, as a result, the more copies you can print for each set-up, such as when you use color, the better off and cheaper the cost per copy will be. A good quality print shop can set this up for you and will quote you prices that can be locked down for the course of a year. The mailing list can be maintained either in-house or using an outside mailing service. The mailing can be done either bulk third class or first class. You will have to check with the post office or the mail service to get the exact procedures. You generally will need over 200 copies in order to take advantage of discounted rates.

Much of what we have talked about in discussing marketing has to do with information and education. A medical practice is very much a professional service and utilizes information in order to act and deliver the service.

The conveyance and reinforcement of good information and good health education equal good patient care. We all know of stories where patients are carefully told the course of action they need to take, the order in which multiple drugs are to be taken, and the like. It is fairly common for patients to immediately forget all this information and instruction as soon as they walk out the door. This is somewhat akin to meeting someone at a party and promptly forgetting his name. Many hospitals will give patients who are discharged from the emergency room an instruction sheet; if a hospital can do that, a physician practice needs to consider doing the same thing. If you have common situations, particularly where information is confusing, it will behoove you to print up common instruction sheets to be given to the patient. Many pharmacies provide written information sheets on prescription drugs. These information sheets include a description of the drug, its actions, possible complications and side effects, interactions with other medications and foods, what to do if the patient forgets to take a dose at the usual time—in short, very helpful, useful information in plain English. A number of specialty societies also produce information brochures that can be readily accessed, as do several commercial providers of books and pamphlets.

Using the Internet to Promote the Practice

The Internet actually has been around for a number of years under various guises, principally designed as a means for researchers at different locations to communicate with each other. The development of "browser" software and the World Wide Web have enabled the introduction of sophisticated graphics and the ability to search through thousands of sites and locations in order to locate relevant information. Those events helped to push the Internet from a simple communication device to a powerful pipeline for communication, capable of linking all parts of the world. The number of people who have access to and use the Internet continues to grow rapidly, and prices for unlimited access through Internet service providers (ISPs) continue to come down. The wealth of information posted for health care professionals is enormous—some of my favorite sites are listed in Appendix F.

How does the Internet fit into *your* marketing strategy? As with many things, it depends upon what you are trying to accomplish. The Internet has several possible applications for a medical practice:

1. E-mail between office, home, hospital, and/or other providers.
2. E-mail between office and patients to handle routine requests (prescription refills) and perhaps questions.
3. A web site for the practice.

A web site offers the most intriguing possibilities for a practice. First, however, assess the degree of use of the Internet by your patients and other providers. A simple means of accomplishing this would be to ask a simple question when patients check in for a visit, such as: "We're conducting a brief survey today. Do you or does anyone living in your home use the Internet on a regular basis? If yes, at home, at work, or both? Thank you."

To date, there are no solid data as to Internet access and usage. Yet, the Internet is a very inexpensive media. While it is true that you can spend tens of thousands of dollars on building a site, you also can build a site by yourself, if you're so inclined, for a few hundred dollars worth of software. In many communities, graphic design firms have developed web site development capabilities and offer reasonable fees. As with anything else, shop around and review samples of other web sites to look for styles that appeal to you.

A basic web site for a practice would include the following information:

I. Home Page

A. Name, address, phone and fax numbers, e-mail address (with hyperlink to "memo" page, enabling the user to write a note and e-mail it directly to the practice).

B. Summary description (one paragraph) of the practice.

C. Contents of the site with hyperlinks to appropriate pages.

II. Physician Page

Biographies / areas of specialization / interest with photos of each physician and midlevel practitioner.

III. "How to Find Us" Page

This is of particular value if you are a specialty practice and do not have ongoing relationships with patients. Ideally, this page should include a map with streets and specific landmarks to aid new patients in finding your office(s).

IV. Frequently Asked Questions (FAQ) Page

These questions should be common ones that do not need to be tailored to a specific individual to be of value to the user. You also might describe certain procedures or tests done in your practice.

V. Prevention Page

Write your own, copy federal publications (with appropriate credit), and / or hyperlink to other sites with prevention information. (See appendix F.)

VI. Making Appointments Page

This page should include your office hours, days when closed, financial policies, managed care plan and other plan participation, and other necessary information to help patients to schedule an appointment for your services.

VII. Prescription Refill Page

This page is an e-mail memo form that patients can complete to request a prescription refill. The requested information should include: name, address, telephone, drug, pharmacy and phone number, and prescription number.

Let patients, other providers, and the general public know that your practice has introduced a web site. Print the web site URL and your e-mail address on all stationery and printed material. Monitor the usage of the site, and survey users of the e-mail, appointment and prescription refill capabilities as to their satisfaction.

Web sites need maintenance and refreshing to be used. Make sure that the information posted is correct and current, and add new features or update information routinely. While I would not necessarily make the setting up a web site a top marketing priority (except in those few markets with heavy concentration of high-tech oriented businesses and residents).

The Role of Preventative Medicine Programs in Promoting the Practice

Many managed care plans have reintroduced the incentives for preventative medicine and an active and aggressive role by primary care physicians in taking the time to educate patients. Some health plans have active preventative medicine programs underway and will pay bonuses to physicians and patients for preventative medicine activities. Some health plans, for example, will pay part of health club memberships and sponsor inexpensive wellness programs, including smoking cessation programs, weight management, and the like.

An excellent single source of information and materials has been produced by the United States Department of Health and Human Services called, "Put Prevention into Practice."[2] The action kit includes a clinician's handbook, personal health guidebooks for physicians and for patients, stickers to be put on the chart to remind the physician to discuss items with the patient, a form for charting the documentation of prevention activities, and the like. Much of the material, since it is produced by the federal government, does not hold a copyright and can be reproduced locally using local printers. Do be aware that some of the material in the handbook does have a copyright from other organizations; and for this material, you will need clearance before using it yourself, or

[2]This action kit can be ordered form the superintendent of Documents for $57. Ask for the "Put Prevention into Practice Education and Action Kit," stock number 017-001-00492-8.

you may need to purchase the material from the copyright owner. While physicians may be aware of many of the recommendations in the clinician's handbook, the value is in putting all of this information together in a step-by-step format that also discusses implementation techniques for a preventative medicine program and preventative medicine protocols and practice.

Critical to any preventative medicine program, obviously, is active patient involvement. The handbook notes that most studies have found that levels of patient interest in preventative services are usually higher than clinicians expect. The handbook notes that some studies have shown that patient or parent-held records, such as those to promote childhood immunizations, are well received by clinicians and patients and are useful in tracking and promoting both child and adult preventative care. The personal health guide and the child health guide included in the action kit have been designed to meet that need and are worth trying. My recommendation is to buy this kit, go through it, start using it in your practice, and see how it best works for you and your patients. Follow up and see how patients like the materials. Additional supplies can be ordered, and note that orders of 100 packages or more of the same item, such as the stickers, flowsheets, reminder postcards, and health guides, are allowed a 25 percent discount when sent to a U.S. address from the Government Printing Office.

As a general rule, any item that you give out to your patients should have your practice's name on it. Preprinted stickers saying "Compliments of Dr. John Smith" with your address and phone number should be attached to every one of the preprinted publications you buy from any source. When you have publications printed yourself, again, your full name, address, and telephone number should be included.

The preventative action kit includes reminder postcards that can be mailed to patients for certain preventative care activities. There is one for adults and one for parents, and these fit into a standard file box. They are folded and stapled for privacy before mailing. A tickler file may be created by addressing the card at the time of the patient's visit and filing it under the month of the next needed visit. Reminder cards can then be mailed at the beginning of the month on a routine basis.

The kit also includes flowsheets for preventative care. There are three sets of templates that can be reproduced: one for adults, one for children, and a separate one for childhood immunizations. There are also instructions for creating practice-specific flowsheets. The self-sticking notes and colored stickers are a prompt for preventative discussions at a visit scheduled for other reasons. Colored alert stickers are permanently placed in a conspicuous location on the outside or inside of the chart to remind clinicians and staff of ongoing preventative care needs such as smoking, alcohol abuse, or lead poisoning. There are 16 different colored stickers, including a blank one provided in the kit. These can either be purchased from the Government Printing Office (GPO) or printed locally. Packs of 500 stickers cost $6.50 from the GPO.

The Role of the Office in Promoting the Practice

The last area of discussion concerning the basics of marketing is the concept of operations as marketing. As we have discussed, you and your office are the practice and you and your office and everything surrounding the office are the service that is provided to your patients, that is, the product. As such, everything you do, from how patients are greeted to staff attitudes, is critical to the success of your practice. Patient satisfaction is governed by the entire visit experience, from the time the patient walks in the door to the time she leaves. One author has suggested the analogy to how one feels on the first day of work at a new job. Being excited, the example goes, is a good thing. Even being nervous can be good. However, if one feels fearful and uneasy, there is a problem.

Patients coming in the door should feel welcome and comfortable in the practice setting. The environment needs to have some warmth in its design, by doing such things as adding plants (which can be artificial), avoiding the use of very bright fluorescent lighting, and, of course, not having the required employee posters in the reception room.

Staff attitudes always need to be upbeat, positive, and very welcoming to patients. The classic example is the Wal-Mart store with a greeter at the front door, something now copied by KMart. A professional service such as medicine is a very personal experience, and a smiling, welcoming greeting sets everything off on a good note. I am personally a fan of calling the room where the patients sit the reception room as opposed to the waiting room. As MGMA's Bette Waddington once pointed out, patients are being received; they are not waiting.

Earlier in this book I've discussed aspects of the practice operations in terms of relating to patients, other physicians, and other providers. My theme is this: Medical practices need to be organized around the needs of the patients. All of the interactions between patients and the practice are part of the service, and all need the same commitment and attention to patients. This is what makes a good medical practice an exceptional practice.

PATIENT SATISFACTION SURVEYS

Managed care plans are placing a great deal of importance on patient satisfaction. Some plans and employers are issuing requests for proposals (RFPs) to select the providers that will be allowed into the network. Among the items being asked for are patient satisfaction studies from the preceding two to three years. If your practice has any patient satisfaction data, this is likely to be an advantage over most other practices. The best way to measure patient satisfaction is through routine surveys of a random sample of patients.

When setting up a patient satisfaction survey, it is important that pointed questions be posed, asking people to rate your practice in terms of convenience, accessibility, responsiveness of the physician and the staff to the needs of the patient, and so on. The questions can be either yes or no, on a scale of one to five, or open ended, in which the respondent is asked to write in her answer. A sound sampling technique of a random selection of patients seen in the office is critical to making this information valuable to you. Anonymity needs to be guaranteed.

One way to do this is to ask every third, fifth, or tenth patient who comes into the office to complete a survey and either leave it at the desk or mail it back in a self-addressed, prepaid envelope. Another method would be to randomly select patients seen in a time period, say a month, and mail them a similar survey. As discussed earlier, telephone surveys may be problematic in terms of confidentiality when conducted by an outside party.

Some examples of questions to be asked in a patient satisfaction questionnaire regard:

- Ease of scheduling appointments and convenience of hours.
- Convenience of location.
- Appearance of office.
- Waiting time.
- Length of time the doctor spent with you.
- Availability after hours.
- Promptness in returning phone calls.
- Friendliness and courtesy extended to you by the staff.
- The doctor's explanations, instructions, and responses to your questions (did you have time to ask all of your questions?)
- Thoroughness and technical skill of the doctor and professional staff.
- Overall quality of care.

Over time, you will see some trends developing. Most importantly, there should be very high levels of being rated excellent or very good. Anything lower than that points out areas of concern. More than 90 percent of your patients should rate you as excellent or very good in most of these areas. If you find areas that are of concern, you also can randomly follow up with pointed, open ended questions focusing on those areas, asking patients for more specific feedback.

Most importantly, in doing a patient satisfaction questionnaire you need to be honest with yourself. It is easy to explain away less than high levels of satisfaction as simply that patients are very tough in their grading, or very demanding or unreasonable, that is, they "don't understand the needs of the practice." This is self-defeating and delusional at best.

Patient satisfaction studies should be an ongoing event. While they need not be conducted on a continuous basis, a sample drawn every six months or every quarter would give you the feedback that you need. The findings should then be compared to previous studies to identify and track any changes, either positive or negative. To facilitate tracking, the same questions need to be used from one survey to the next.

A local market research firm should be able to design and implement a survey for you. The Medical Group Management Association has materials for sale that will be useful. There are also several companies that are marketing surveys, and offer to compare findings (anonymously) with those of other clients, thereby providing a benchmark for comparison.

EVALUATING YOUR MARKETING STRATEGY

To make a marketing program work, the first thing you need to do is figure out what sorts of marketing you are already doing. You will find that you have, in fact, undertaken a number of marketing efforts, even though you may not think of it as that. Your first task, then, is to audit yourself, looking at current activities, accomplishments, and areas of concern. Current activities include all advertising, including yellow pages advertising and the must-do advertising, how your telephone is answered, how your staff greets people, publications and patient education materials, and your patient satisfaction survey. Your first survey should include a relatively large sample will serve as the basis for devising and implementing a marketing plan.

Other parties who should be surveyed include your office staff and other physicians and professional customers, including the hospital, labs, imaging centers, and other professional services with which you interact. The object here is to find some feedback as to how you interact with your colleagues and how you can better help them do their job. An example of this is how timely referral letters are written. If you are a primary care physician, are patients referred to a specialist with the proper paperwork, particularly the referral form? Are patients sent back to the referring practice? Are patient appointments made on a timely basis? Can the other offices get through to you on your phone lines? Are pages and phone calls returned promptly?

As part of the audit, look at any advertising you already have been doing, must-do ads, and placements in newspapers, magazines, or on the radio. Look at what you have done on a month-by-month basis over the past 12 months, including any special mailings to patients as well as routine mailings. Also look at your patient communication materials, including all forms that a patient sees, and evaluate them in terms of quality, clarity, and readability. This also includes your bills and their comprehensiveness and readability. Your next step then is to develop a marketing plan.

1. Identify your goals. What are you trying to achieve in terms of increased revenue, increased patient flow, increased geographic area, or prestige?
2. Plan specific activities to address each goal.
3. Set time frames to achieve each of these goals and measure your progress by year, quarter, and month.
4. Adopt terms of measurement, such as, increased awareness, increased visits and increased number of patients, and increased referrals.

The marketing plan must clearly state the objectives of increased visibility and awareness, reputation, increased market share and visit volume. Its implementation needs to specifically state what activities will be undertaken. For example, your plan may outline these activities:

- Run six radio spots in rotation on four stations: all news, rock, country, and classical.
- Provide an interview regarding flu shots on one television news segment.
- Run one ad each Sunday in the business and television sections.
- Run one ad each week in the style section.
- Insert a response card in low country magazine for a flu shot brochure.

In Appendix D is The Medical Practice Business Plan Workbook, and there I've laid out some of the data to collect and some of the goals to identify for your practice in developing and implementing a marketing plan. It's easy to spend money on marketing, but in doing so, always find a way to measure whether you are achieving a marketing goal. How many people attended the corn roast you helped sponsor? How many read the church bulletin you advertise in? How many health information brochures did you give out at the health fair? How many people first heard of you when you spoke at the mall walking club meeting, and they're now a patient?

10 CHAPTER

Creating Change

Now we have come full circle, having looked at what is changing, why it's changing, how it's changing, and how you are changing. It's time, then, to turn our attention to making change happen. There are dozens of books and "how to" publications available in various forms and formats out there that you can consult for advice regarding how to create change, so forgive me if some of what is written here sounds familiar. With it all, there are many insights that can provide insight and advice for the physician practice.

Even though change is natural and ever present in people's lives, people and organizations resist change the way a body fights disease. General Colin Powell, commenting on his time as a White House Fellow at the Office of Management and Budget, observed that it can take two years for an order from the president to be implemented in the bureaucracy. Even in a small organization, the staff can resist change to the point of exasperation of the manager or even the owner. Resistance can be open, such as refusal to follow a new procedure. Or resistance can be more subtle and insidious when accomplished through a passive means—hiding how a report was prepared, ignoring instructions and continuing to do something the old way, starting on a project but never quite completing it, and making end runs around the manager trying to implement change and encouraging the owners or superiors to override the manager.

Why do physician practices need to change? Why did I write this book, why did Irwin Professional Publishing choose to publish it, and why did you buy it? Because medical practices are facing the ultimate threat to a business: we are being thrust into a new and different business. We used to be a professional practice providing the professional service of medical care. We now are in the business of managing premium dollars, acting as the agent buying healthcare services for the buyer, the health plan or employer, who turns around and presents the services to its members and employees. Our customers of old are no longer our customers; instead, we are selling to a new buyer group that is making the purchasing decisions for large numbers of people and is suspicious of our motivations, skills and capabilities, and the ultimate value of the service itself.

So we must transform ourselves in order to survive. Some physicians—well, actually a whole lot of physicians—are committing euthanasia on the practice by closing it down, merging with another group, or selling to a hospital or physician practice management company. Some are still in the denial stage. Some are paralyzed by indecision. Others are aggressively changing and transforming. Whatever route is chosen, change and transform the physician will.

I sometimes think that the change process is like the stages of grieving. When I do my seminars on managed care, I frequently will have a physician in the group who starts to argue that managed care organizations (MCOs) interfere with needed care, are hurting patients, that the quality of care and outcome indicators have no meaning, and so on. I'm only the messenger, conveying what is happening and offering strategies to successfully deal with MCOs and the new health care environment. I encounter the stages of anger and even denial frequently. I can only urge these physicians, and the reader, to work toward at least a partial acceptance stage.

> When you tell them what, you get their hands and maybe their heads, but when you tell them why, you get their hearts.
>
> *Dutch chief executive*[1]

---

[1]As quoted in Litwin, Bray, and Brooke, *Mobilizing the Corporation: Bringing Strategy to Life* (Englewood Cliffs, NJ: Prentice Hall, 1996).

Until this point, this book has focused on the nitty gritty, practical strategies and techniques for medical practices in the changing business of healthcare. But to accomplish many of these changes requires the organization itself to change. Organizations have personalities, just like people—here, we call it the "culture" of the organization.

The Purrington Foundation has done some very interesting work in developing a focused approach to change. Much of this can be accessed via its web site (www.mobilze.com) and book (see footnote). Many of the ideas presented in the following discussion are based upon this work. I've made my own adaptations and interpretations.

In earlier chapters, I suggested that all organizations can be viewed in terms of four resources: human, physical, financial, and information and technology. But when looking at an organization as a functioning system, there are different aspects to look at, which Litwin calls the four cardinals:

- *Purpose* is the brain of the organization, the why, the psychological state.
- *Infrastructure* is the musculoskeletal system, where purpose is translated into form.
- *Guidance* is the day-to-day direction, inspiration, and feedback—the "management" of the enterprise.
- *Resources* is the how the change gets accomplished.

Change in a practice means a change in the purpose and/or a change in the infrastructure of the practice. Change happens because of a change in the guidance. Change is accomplished by a change in the *resources*—more and/or different resources, or resources that themselves change.

Go back to the last paragraph, second sentence: change happens because of a change in the guidance. In the end, it all comes back to management, the management of the practice.

> Whenever something happens, it's because of a megalomaniac with a mission.
>
> *Unknown, quoted by Tom Peters*

---

[2]See Litwin, Bray, and Brooke, *Mobilizing the Organization: Bringing Strategy to Life* (Englewood Cliffs, NJ: Prentice Hall, 1996).

For change to happen, for your practice to transform itself into an organization that can compete and succeed in the health care industry environment of today, the physician owners or directors must come to decide that change they will. Without the symbolism of words and the example of actions, all the business and strategic plans in the world will be worthless—another tree dying for the sins of bad management.

> You manage stability, you lead change.
>
> *Dutch executive*

The Purrington thesis uses the term "guidance" as the descriptor of the principal role of top management. I like it because it fits my own thesis for implementing strategy in an organization: Strategy must be articulated and communicated throughout the organization, so that all understand the purpose and direction of the organization. Litwin describes guidance as developing a "natural navigation system," so that the strategy and purpose of the organization are imbued in the culture.

The guidance of an organization involves more than mission statements, motivational posters, and meetings. Guidance happens day-to-day—in the hallway discussion, the staff meeting, the performance evaluation, the encouragement and approval for outside training programs and conferences, the debate over issues and decisions. I may be stealing a quote in saying, Strategy is made in the boardroom, but it is implemented on the factory floor.

Change is very difficult for people; people need stability and few seek the risk and the unknown of change. Organizational change impacts relationships, destabilizes the routine of work, imposes new sets of standards and expectations, and impacts employees' ability to earn a living.

Achieving a new culture requires leadership, a leadership that ultimately must come from the physicians. All of the physician owners must agree to and commit themselves to the changes that are to be implemented. The staff will be looking to the physicians to set an example and the example the physicians set in words and in deeds will be what tells the staff what is important to change. Behavior, attitudes, and actions that are rewarded—or that go unpunished—are what will communicate the new culture and strategy of the practice. Bob Nelson has developed the Twelve Cs of Change?[3]

1. *Clarity:* Why the business needs to change.
2. *Consistency:* Clear objectives .
3. *Context:* Connect the changes being made to something else, such as outside forces.
4. *Colleagues:* Get others on your side.
5. *Champions:* The people who create and lead the changes.
6. *Communication:* Tell everyone what and why.
7. *Commitment:* Are the leaders behind the changes?
8. *Celebration:* Celebrate and reward successes, even small ones.
9. *Coalitions:* Relate to other parts of the organization or outside firms you do business with, such as other practices, hospitals, and health plans.
10. *Consequences:* Describe and project what it will be like after the changes are accomplished.
11. *Cement:* When the changes are in place and fine-tuned, fix them into the "system."
12. *Courage:* Have the guts to do it.

With all this said, how do you make this happen? Through training. By training, I mean more than the time that is spent teaching technical skills. Training is any educational activity that enhances the ability of an employee to do his job and helps the organization accomplish its mission. Time set aside for training can be as short as five minutes or as long as a weekend retreat (and yes, sometimes longer). Through this training, the leadership can communicate to the rest of the organization the changes desired. In addition, it can reward the successes, discuss the failures, and invigor the staff into continuing to move forward. The message must be clear, consistent, communicated daily in many small ways, and reinforced through the system of evaluating performance and rewards.

---

[3] This checklist is taken from Litwin, Bray, and Brooke, *Mobilizing the Corporation: Bringing Strategy to Life* (Englewood Cliffs, NJ: Prentice-Hall, 1996).

For any practice, no matter how small, a regular meeting of all the staff members should be held no less than once a month. Set a time limit of one hour, perhaps during a lunch hour. (Staff would have to be paid for the meeting time and, if held during the lunch hour, bringing in sandwiches or pizza would be a nice touch.) The format of the meeting should be very informal. To lead off, the managing physician or practice administrator might bring staff up to date on things such as: managed care plan activity, practice visit volumes, accounts receivable (A/R), and expenses. You don't need to give out all of the details if you don't want to, but many the staff will already know about your financial situation and having this information will put other actions in perspective. I worked at a hospital many years ago where the entire staff—all the way through housekeeping and laundry—asked about the census, for each employee knew that (at the time) that was the key indicator of the hospital's success, financial condition . . . and his job.

Other points to note during this "update" include any forthcoming marketing activities. If you have planned radio announcements, or whatever, make sure that the staff knows about it before it happens. Are you using ad specialties (giveaways)? Make sure that the staff is given them, too. The members of your staff are your best marketers, and they are very much a part of what physicians do. Their care and feeding is a top priority for management attention.

I've been discussing how to convey change, but let me step back and discuss *what* to change. I believe that for many practices the first thing to do is to determine a purpose for the organization. It may be as simple as medical care for patients, but your practice also may commit to research, to a subspecialty, to being active in public health activities in the community, and to education, prevention, or clinical education. A statement of purpose needs to be clear, concise, and understandable to the staff and patients. Flowery language is not necessary and can be counterproductive.

Now, the hard part: you had better mean what you say and be prepared to act on what you have written. The fastest way to destroy credibility and damage your practice is to put out a poetic, inspiring mission statement that is antithetical to the behavior of the physicians and the staff. For example, a statement of purpose that states a commitment to a caring and supportive atmosphere is rendered a sham when staff members don't smile in greeting a patient, are slow about answering or returning phone calls, or generate bills that are indecipherable. A physician can promptly destroy the message by complaining about patient calls or instructing staff to schedule Medicaid and HMO patients late in the afternoon or during other inconvenient times.

> Nobody was ever motivated by a number.
>
> *Jack Welch, Chairman, General Electric*

I believe that most of the people in health care are here because they want to help people, and they basically like people. I believe that we have allowed too many bad habits, practices, and attitudes to permeate our hospitals and offices, and we have ended up passing these on to the next generation. I worked with a hospital client whose house staff had a reputation for being lazy. The house staff had developed an elaborate scoring system for new admissions at night, so that no resident had to do any more admissions and workups than any other. A patient, then, would be admitted to one service at night and then promptly transferred to another service the next morning. By the way, this meant physically moving the patient, because House Staff Law (as in Murphy's Law) read that, "House staff doesn't climb stairs." It got so bad that one night a patient was refused admission from the ER, but was promptly slapped in CCU by another hospital a few hours later.

How was this allowed to happen? How was this allowed to continue? Because this organization and its leadership allowed it. The systems were not written down, but the climate rewarded and failed to punish the behavior.

Author Kurt Lewen defines climate by the equation:[4]

$$B = f(P, E)$$

Where

B = Individual behavior
P = The person
E = The environment

Behavior is a function of the person and the environment.

---

[4] See Litwin, Bray, and Brooke, *Mobilizing the Organization: Bringing Strategy to Life,* (Englewood Cliffs, NJ: Prentice-Hall, 1996).

Let me suggest, then, a standard of behavior—the culture—for a physician practice in the 1990s:

1. Willingness to listen to patients, family, staff, quality assurance practitioners, and others.
2. Curiosity as to "How am I doing?"
3. Dedication to seeking out the "best practices" in terms of cost and outcome.
4. Recommitment to service to patients and a personal physician–patient relationship.
5. Commitment to work cooperatively with other physicians and with their own staffs.
6. Willingness to support, train, educate, and reward—to appreciate—their staff.
7. Commitment to be more open and forthcoming with patients and families about options, pros and cons, and expectations.
8. Willingness to answer for actions and be judged by others.
9. Curiosity as to the financial implications of decisions.
10. Desire to learn about the emotional and moral implications of decisions.

Much of this book has dealt with the infrastructure of the practice and how the organization and procedures can change—and need to change. Many of the changes discussed will happen only with the leadership, commitment, and guidance of the physicians.

Lastly, we turn to resources as the means of making the changes happen. While it is true that to create change you need to change people, notice the statement reads "change people," not "change *the* people." When an organization is being changed, the people in it must be changed, that is, their attitudes, the methods and behaviors they use in doing tasks, and how they interrelate and interact with colleagues, patients, and other healthcare providers. It would not be unusual to find that many people want to make these changes, but they lack the ability, the authority, the sense of permission—the safety—to do it. I worked in an organization where a new CEO unleashed years of pent up ideas simply by constantly telling us, "Just do it!"

Changing behavior and unleashing your staff when the behavior and expectations of the leader have changed dramatically make guidance critical; the leaders must be constantly among the "troops," supporting and encouraging their efforts and ideas and commending them for actions taken. In the 12 Cs of change described above, number 8 is "celebrate." So celebrate success, celebrate effort. By doing so publicly, having the staff tell others how they accomplished a difficult task or goal, other colleagues are educated as to what is possible, how it is possible, and what kind of recognition they will receive for doing it.

Tom Peters tells the story of a motor pool and maintenance division in the U.S. Army. The officer in charge turned the organization around, cutting down time, improving reliability, and so on. And the officer did it, Peters tells us, by celebrating success. How does the army celebrate? It has a parade. What did this officer do? He had a parade. Trucks, jeeps, all the motor pool stuff went rumbling by, complete with a band, flags, and commendations. Families, friends, and other units were all invited to watch and cheer.

A hospital where I worked hadn't held an employee award dinner in several years; it just lapsed for various reasons, partly due to lack of interest. When it was revived, however, one thing that was noticed was the longevity of the staff. The Sunday after the dinner, we placed a full-page ad in the local paper, in the main section, saluting staff members with five or more years of service and *listing every single name!* It was the smartest thing we had ever done. The family, friends, and neighbors of our employees all saw the ad and commented on it, and our people felt enormous pride. Imagine being an employee, working perhaps in a low skill job, opening the paper one morning and seeing a full page ad with your name in it.

Unfortunately, the process of changing an organization is peculiar to each organization. I've tried in this chapter to lay out some guidance and rules but, in the end, it's up to you as the practice leaders and managers.

Some final advice:

- Some people will never "get it." They may need to go. As Robert Kennedy once said, "Twenty percent of the people will be against anything."

- Start by creating and making the case for change—what threats, events, and opportunities are behind your action?
- Clearly lay out where you want to go.
- Take care to reassure and support people on the "me" issues. As Robert Frost once said, "There's nothing I'm afraid of like scared people."
- Get people involved in the solution—let them experiment, let them fail, and be proud when they truly succeed, because they will.
- Be there—walk around a lot, talk to people, listen to gripes, be a friend and a leader.
- Defuse fear.
- Celebrate.

APPENDICES

APPENDIX A

Due Diligence Checklist

1. Name of organization: ____________________
2. Type of relationship: HMO ____ PPO ____ Network___ IPA ___ Other________________
3. History (when founded, where?):

   ____
4. Ownership / form of organization:

   ____
5. Local and corporate officers:

   Chief executive officer (CEO): ____________________

   Chief operation officer (COO): ____________________

   Corporate chief provider relations officers: ___________

   Chief regional executive: ____________________

   Regional marketing executive: ____________________

   Regional provider relations director: ______________

   Regional medical director: ____________________

   Regional utilization review: ____________________

   Regional claims management representative: ___________
6. Copy of agreement, including all references attachments and exhibits.
7. Proposed fee schedule.
8. Copy of latest financial statement. If public corporation, request "investor packet" to include Form 10-K.
9. Current provider network in your market (if existing plan).
10. List of major employer groups in your market.
11. Reference checks with at least five providers from local (if applicable) and nonlocal markets.

12. Discussion of marketing plan: geographic areas to be targeted, employer groups, projected enrollment in years one, two, and three.
13. Opportunities for designation as an exclusive or preferred provider for certain services.
14. Claim billing system:

    HCFA 1500/UB 92 ______

    Physicians: RBRV system ______ CPT coding ______

    Is a different or supplemental coding system used? If yes, obtain copy and provide explanations.

    Availability of electronic billing ______

    Electronic remittance______

    Guaranteed payment cycle ______
    Is there designated contact person for billing problems?

    ____

    Are there direct and toll-free numbers for billing issues?

    ____
15. Referrals: Is primary care clearance required? Method of documentation: ____________________________
16. Services requiring prior approval:

    By primary care physician?_______________

    By plan medical director? __________________
17. Grievance procedures, penalties for noncompliance:
18. Procedures for out-of-plan approval:
19. Documentation provided (i.e., manuals, newsletters, meetings, etc.):

20. Required procedures that vary from your current procedures:

a. ____________________

b. ____________________

c. ____________________

d. ____________________

e. ____________________

Assess impact on operations:

____

____

21. Quality and utilization review procedures, requirements, etc.

22. Copies of marketing materials and information given to members and prospective members.

23. Confirmed conversations/explanations (in writing).

24. Review of indemnification and hold harmless clauses (understand implications and notify your liability carriers or self insured plan administrator).

25. Obtain final legal review.

APPENDIX B

Sample Reference Check on MCOs

1. How long have you had a contract with MCO________?
2. What reimbursement mechanism is used?

   Discounted fee for service _____ Risk Pool _____

   Capitation _____ Other _____

   (*Warning: Do not discuss specific fees, particularly in your market area!*)
3. Was the MCO's staff open to discussing the terms of the contract?
4. What level representative did you work with on the contract?
5. Was a copy of the contract and fee schedule offered?
6. Did the MCO provide you with utilization or actuarial data?
7. Does the MCO appear to be fair in its dealings with your organization?
8. Did the MCO appear to be fair in its dealings with your patients?
9. If you felt that you had a choice, would you renew a contract with the MCO?

APPENDIX C

MCO Contracting Action Plan

1. Identify all MCOs operating in your market:

   Name: ______________________

   Address: ______________________________

   Tel: ____________ Fax: ________________

   Administrative Director: ______________________

   Medical Director: ________________________

   Provider Relations Director: ____________________

   # covered lives ______________

   Areas (counties) licensed to operate: _________________

Sources for data: Interstudy, state insurance and health departments, state HMO trade organization, colleagues, phone book, news articles.

2. Identify all MCOs operating within 50-mile radius and in nearest major metropolitan area. Collect same data as in #1.
3. Compile public information concerning above: new articles, annual reports, SEC filings, regulatory filings.
4. Prepare health plan fee schedule comparative worksheet. For capitation rates, compare to fee for service rates (full and discounted).
5. Conduct cost study of key services.
6. Collect credentialing information on all licensed professionals: C.V., copies of diplomas, transcripts, board certifications, malpractice insurance, reference letters, etc. For those materials where a separate request must be made for each credentialing process, compile all addresses and fees for each organization.

7. Determine utilization by service / code by payer, by age group, by sex. Determine utilization rates for each and note variations, developing a "range" of utilization rates by service / code.
8. Conduct satisfaction studies:

   _____ Overall organization.

   _____ Physicians / clinicians.

   _____ Nursing staff.
9. Conduct quality-of-care review. Use NCQA guidelines as starting point:

   _____ Patient access.

   _____ Preventive care.

   _____ Utilization of services.
10. Compile outcome data and information. Examples:

    _____ Readmission rates.

    _____ Reoccurrence rates.

    _____ 5-year survivability.

    _____ Low birthweight.

    _____ ER visits / admission rates.
11. Development, adoption, and use of internal clinical guidelines, care maps, etc.
12. Risk management issues: major and minor adverse events.

© 1996 Lucash & Company. This is a sample action plan presented as a basis for adaptation by the user to the particular needs and circumstances presented.

Medical Practice Business Plan Workbook

I. Background of Practice (History, where / when founded, growth milestones, etc.)

____

____

____

II. Form of Business Organization

A. _____PC/PA _____LLC/LLP _____ "C" Corp
_____ Partnership _____Sole Proprietorship

B. Advantages of current form of organization:

____

____

C. Disadvantages of current form of organization:

____

____

III. Management

A. Owners / shareholders:

____

____

B. Managing physician:

____

____

C. Administrator:

____

____

© 1996 Lucash & Company. All Rights Reserved.

D. Business manager / chief financial officer:

____

____

E. Chief operations officer:

____

____

F. Management structure (include table of organization):

____

____

____

____

Assessment of Management Skills

Management Skills	Above Average	Adequate	Assistance Needed	Education Needed
Accounting				
Planning				
Contracting/negotiation				
Organization				
Financial management				
People management				
Sales/business development				
Managed care				
Clinical management				
Decision making				
Personnel policies				
Pricing				
Board				
Marketing				

G. How does practice compensate in area where management is lacking?

____

____

____

____

H. Advisors to the practice:

1. Legal: ______________________________
2. Accounting: __________________________
3. Tax: ________________________________
4. Marketing: __________________________
5. Retirement plan management: ____________
6. Retirement plan investment management: ______

Assessment of Advisors

	Responsiveness	Value	Understanding of Business	Confidentiality	Quality
Legal					
Accountant					
Tax					
Marketing					
Retirement Plan Management					
Retirement Plan Investment Management					

IV. Technical Staff

A. Employee physicians:

____

____

B. Employee midlevel practitioners:

___

___

C. Technical staff:

___

___

Assessment of Technical Staff

Management Skills	Above Average	Adequate	Assistance Needed	Education Needed
Organization				
People management				
Sales				
Clinical management				
Decision making				
Effectiveness				
Ethics				
Professionalism				
Technical skills				
Clinical skills/knowledge				

V. Support Staff

	Technical Knowledge	Patient Relations	Relations w/ Staff	Organizational Skills	Decision Making Skills
Reception					
Billing office					
Medical assistants					
Scheduling					

VI. Key Business Relationships

A. Hospital(s):

____

B. Top 10 referring physicians:

____

C. Physicians referred to by specialty:

____

____

____

____

D. Home health:

____

E. Laboratory:

____

F. Rehabilitation:

____

G. Imaging:

____

H. Other:

____

____

VII. Key Contacts

A. MCOs:

____

B. Chamber of Commerce:

____

C. Bank:

____

D. Political officials:

____

E. Medical society:

____

F. Hospital(s):

____

G. IPA(s):

____

H. PHO(s):

____

VIII. Personnel

A. Needed employee skills:

____

____

B. How to achieve:

_____In-house _____Seminars _____Conferences

_____Books/manuals

____

____

C. New positions:

____

____

D. Sources of employees:

____

____

E. Written personnel policies:

____

____

IX. Services

A. Office visits:

____

B. Hospital visits:

____

C. Testing/treatment (list):

____

D. Imaging:

____

X. Customers

A. *Major employers:*

____

____

____

____

B. *List all MCOs:*

1. Number of members __________

2. Age of business __________

3. Number of years in local market __________

4. Number of employers / major employers

____

C. *Patients:*

1. Run report for each zip code:
   - *a.* Number of patients
   - *b.* Age distribution
   - *c.* Sex
   - *d.* Payer
2. Utilization of principal services
3. Potential customers by above parameters by zip code
4. Create map of market area showing primary and secondary service areas
5. Average utilization by patient ____________
6. Average cost of services per patient ____________
7. Average charges per patient ____________
8. Average collections per patient ____________

XI. Location / Facility

A. Appearance

____

____

B. Future prospects of location

____

____

C. Annual cost (rent / mortgage / depreciation)

____

____

D. Utility cost

____

____

E. Maintenance and repairs

____

____

F. Insurance

____

____

G. Other costs

____

____

H. Capital improvements needed in next three years

____

____

XII. Competitor Analysis

A. Location

____

____

B. Number of physicians

____

____

C. MCO contracts

____

____

D. Direct contracts

____

____

E. Testing/procedure capabilities

____

____

F. Image/reputation

____

____

G. Hospital affiliations

____

____

H. Appearance

____

____

I. Availability

____

____

J. Management

____

____

K. Stability

____

____

L. Advertising/marketing

____

____

M. Other

____

____

XIII. Marketing Strategy

A. What business are we in?

B. Findings of patient satisfaction study.

C. Findings of referring physician satisfaction study.
D. Findings of quality-of-care indicators report from MCO.
E. Marketing strategy:
  1. Who are we trying to reach?
    MCOs ______________________

    ____

    Employers ______________________

    ____

    Politicians ______________________

    ____

    Patients ______________________

    ____

    Others ______________________

    ____

  2. How do we reach them?:

    ____

    ____

  3. Check off which media are to be used for promotion of each major service:

Media	Service A	Service B	Service C
Radio			
Television			
Over air			
Cable only			
Newspaper			
Direct mail			
Yellow pages			
Shopper (*Pennysaver*)			
Billboard/outside			
Seminars			
Magazine			
Health fairs			
Promotional items			
Other			

F. Image:

Characteristic	Superior	Above Average	Average	Below Average	Poor
Quality-of-care					
Up-to-date/leading edge					
Caring atmosphere					
Bedside manner					
Responsiveness to phone calls, questions					
Staff attitude					
Access/parking					
Other					

G. Areas of advantage over competition:

____

____

H. Areas of weakness as compared to competition:

____

____

I. Areas of competitive activity:

____

____

J. Describe image you wish to achieve:

____

____

K. Describe the steps you will take to support this image:

____

____

L. Advertising theme:

____

____

XIV. Financial

A. Assess changes in revenue by service line for past two calendar years or latest available 12-month period:

Revenue By Service	Last Year	This Year	Change	% Change	Projected Revenue
Service A					
Service B					
Total					

B. Prepare schedules of key overhead expenses:

1. Personnel register:
All positions are designated by position title and control number.

Position	Control Number	FT/PT	Employee Name/Vacant	Scheduled Hours	Pay Rate/ Hour	Total Pay

2. Schedule of insurance:

Policy Type	Value/Limits	Carrier	Agent/Broker	Renewal	Date	Premium
Worker's comp						
Property						
General liability						
Professional liability						
Employee health						
Others (specify)						

3. Schedule of leases:

Type	Amount/Month	Lease Date	End Date	Renew or Return
Facility				
Computers				
Treadmill				
X-ray				
	Total/Month			

C. Projected expenses statement:

Expense by Account	Last Year	This Year	Change	% Change	Projected Expense
Salaries (from schedule)					
Insurance (from schedule)					
List by account					
Total					

D. Compile projected revenue statement and projected expense statement into one combined profit and loss statement, aka, budget:

	Jan	Feb	Mar	Qtr 1	Apr	May	Jun	Qtr 2	Jul	Aug	Sep	Qtr 3	Oct	Nov	Dec	Qtr 4	Total
Revenue																	
Expenses																	
Net income																	

E. Revenue by payer relationships:

Type of Payer	Gross Revenue	Collections	Other (Copay, bonuses)	Total Collections	Collection Rate %
HMO A					
HMO B					
Total					

XV. Action Plan

A. Physician(s) to be recruited: ______________________

____

B. Staff to be recruited: ______________________________

____

C. Training plan:

1. To enhance management skills:

____

____

2. To enhance clinical/technical skills:

____

____

D. Advertising/marketing plan:

____

____

E. Facilities:

____

____

F. Equipment:

____

____

G. Service enhancements, additions, or subtractions:

____

____

H. Consultants / advisors:

____

____

I. Business development activities:

____

____

APPENDIX E

Glossary

Agency for Healthcare Policy and Research (AHCPR) The agency of DHHS that is responsible for developing standards (Conquest 1.0) for the quality, appropriateness, and effectiveness of healthcare services.

Administrative Service Organizations (ASO) Organizations that provide administrative services to support that management of full risk capitation contracts. As examples, ASOs would process and pay claims submitted by other providers.

Alternative Site Provider (ASP) Any provider other than the traditional hospital, medical practice, and outpatient settings. Includes home care, specialty services, birthing centers, ambulatory surgery centers, outpatient mental health, and such.

Capitation A payment system whereby providers are paid a defined payment for a defined scope of services for a defined population set (covered lives) for a defined period of time. Payment is made on the basis of the number of members each month (see PMPM).

Case Management The process by which all matters related to the medical care for a patient are planned, managed, and coordinated by a physician, nurse, or other professional. Case management is intended to ensure continuity and coordination of services, whether inpatient, outpatient, or at home. The goal is to match the appropriate mix and intensity of services with the patient's needs over time.

Closed Panel Usually refers to a group or staff HMO model, where the physicians providing services only provide services for the one HMO, either as employees or under an exclusive contractual basis.

Co-insurance A cost-sharing requirement under health insurance policies, including many HMO and other managed care plans, whereby the insured is responsible for paying a portion or percentage of the costs of covered services after the deductible is paid.

Community Rating The setting of insurance rates based on the average cost of providing health services to all people in a geographic area, without adjusting for each individual's medical history or likelihood of using medical services.

Conquest 1.0 Quality of care standards developed by the Agency for Healthcare Policy and Research of DHHS. First issued in 1996.

Copayment A type of cost-sharing under most HMO and other managed care plans whereby the insured pays a specified flat dollar amount to the provider, usually each time a service is sought.

Credentialing The process of reviewing a practitioners credentials, i.e., training, experience, or demonstrated ability, for the purpose of determining if clinical privileges are to be granted.

Deductible The out-of-pocket expenses that must be paid by the insured before the health plan benefits begin to pay.

Diagnosis-related groups (DRG) A system used by Medicare and other insurers to classify illnesses according to diagnosis and treatment.

Direct Contracting A system whereby an employer or employer group contracts with a network of providers without using a health plan or insurance company. All contracts are between the employer(s) and provider(s), and all claims and payments are transacted between these two parties.

Employee Retirement and Income Security Act (ERISA) The federal law that governs all employee benefit plans, including pension plans and health plans.

Exclusive Provider Organization (EPO) A managed care organization that is organized similarly to PPOs in that providers do not share risk, but requires patients to use network providers in order to receive any of the plan's benefits.

Exclusivity Clause A part of a contract which designates the contracted provider as the sole source of providing certain services to the health plan's insured.

Experience Rating A system where an insurance company evaluates the risk of an individual or the members of a group by looking at the applicant's age, sex, and health history and setting premiums based on those factors.

Fee-for-service The traditional payment method whereby patients pay providers for the services rendered.

Fee Schedule A comprehensive listing of fees used by either a healthcare plan or the government to reimburse physicians and/or other providers on a fee-for-service basis.

Fiscal Intermediary (FI) The agent that has been contracted by Medicare or a health plan to process claims for reimbursement. The intermediary may perform other functions such as provider relations, member relations, education, and such.

Formulary The list of pharmaceuticals and supplies which will be covered by a health plan.

Gatekeeper The role of the primary care physician (PCP) to oversee and coordinate all aspects of a patient's medical care. All services by any provider other than the PCP must be authorized by the PCP.

Group Insurance Any insurance policy or health services contract by which a group of employees and eligible dependents are covered under a single policy or contract issued to their employer or other group entity.

Group Model HMO An HMO that contracts with a multispecialty medical group to provide services for the HMO's members.

Health Maintenance Organization (HMO) HMOs are insurance plans that offer prepaid, comprehensive health coverage for healthcare services, including hospital, physician, and usually prescription drug and vision care, home care, and other services. There is often a sharing of the financial risk of the cost of the services to be provided.

Health Plan Employer Data and Information Set (HEDIS) A set of performance measures designed to standardize the way health plans report data to employers and employees. HEDIS currently measures 5 major areas in 75 standards of health plan performance: quality, access and patient satisfaction, membership and utilization, finance, and descriptive information on health plan management. HEDIS version 3.0 was issued in July 1996.

Hold Harmless Clause A clause in the contract with the MCO whereby the MCO and the physician agree not to hold the other liable for malpractice or corporate malfeasance if either of the parties is found to be liable. Hold Harmless Clauses also refer to the stipulation, often governed by state law, whereby the provider can only seek payment from the MCO—the provider cannot seek payment from the patient unless it is for services that are not covered by the benefits of the plan.

Indemnify To make good a loss.

Indemnification Clause The section of a MCO contract that determines whether one party to the contract will "indemnify" the other party against claims and liability for damages resulting from a legal action against the other party.

Independent Practice Association (IPA) A group of providers, typically just physicians, who organize into a corporation that in turn contracts with HMOs. The IPA may be a "captive IPA," formed solely to contract with one HMO. Some IPAs are now taking on utilization management, practice management, and other roles, as well as accepting and managing "full-risk" capitation contracts.

Managed Care A system that provides for the coordination of health services encompassing the early intervention to control price, volume, delivery site, and intensity of health services provided in order to maximize the health of the insured, and, the goal of which is to maximize the value of health benefits.

Managed Care Organization (MCO) Any organization that provides or claims to provide managed care services—HMOs, PPOs, etc.

Management Services Organization (MSO) An organization formed to manage the nonclinical functions of physician practices, including personnel (whom the MSO may employ), finance, marketing, purchasing, facilities management, MIS, and contracting. (See Physician Practice Management Companies.)

Market The potential customers for a product or service. The market for a service can be defined in terms of geography, industry, demographics, or other means of commonality among potential customers.

Market Share That part of the market potential that an organization has captured; usually market share is expressed as a percentage of the market potential.

Medically Necessary Those covered services required to protect and enhance the health status of a patient that is in accordance with "accepted" standards of medical practice.

Multispecialty Group A group of doctors who represent various medical specialties and who work together in a group practice.

National Committee for Quality Assurance (NCQA) A nonprofit organization created to improve patient care quality and health plan performance in partnership with managed care plans, purchasers, consumers, and the public sector.

Network Model HMO An HMO that contracts with two or more independent group practices to provide health services.

Outcomes Management A system for assessing and identifying preferred medical or surgical intervention or nonintervention that leads to a desired clinical outcome.

Outlier One who does not fall within the norm.

Outpatient Services Outpatient services are medical and other services provided by a hospital or other qualified facility, such as a mental health clinic, rural health clinic, mobile X-ray unit, or free-standing dialysis unit. Such services include outpatient physical therapy services, diagnostic X-ray, and laboratory tests.

Participating Provider A healthcare provider who participates through a contractual arrangement with a healthcare plan, and agrees to accept the plan's fees and comply with certain rules as detailed in the contract.

Physician Hospital Organization A corporation formed by a hospital and its medical staff to contract with MCOs. Typically, the board of directors is shared equally by the hospital and medical staff members. Physicians who join the PHO must make an investment that is "at risk."

Physician Practice Management Company (PPMC) The name being applied to for profit, publicly-traded MSO companies. Examples include: MedPartners and Phycor.

PMPM Per Member Per Month. The dollar amount paid to the provider each month for each person for which the provider is responsible for providing services. This is the basis by which MCOs pay providers under capitation.

PMPY Average cost of providing service for each member each year.

Point-of-Service Plan (POS) Also known as an open-ended HMO, POS plans allow plan members to use non-network providers at their discretion. Members choosing to go "out-of-network" will incur higher out-of-pocket costs than would be the case if a "network" provider was used.

Preferred Provider Organization (PPO) A PPO is a healthcare arrangement between purchasers of care (e.g., employers, insurance companies) and providers that provides benefits at a reduced price by providing members incentives (such as lower deductibles and copays) to use providers within the network. Members who prefer to use nonpreferred physicians may do so, but will incur higher out-of-pocket costs. Preferred providers must agree to specified fee schedules in exchange for a preferred status and are required to comply with certain utilization review guidelines.

Preauthorization A method of monitoring and controlling utilization by evaluating the need for medical service prior to it being performed.

Quality Assurance (QA) Activities and programs intended to assure the quality of care in a defined medical setting. Such programs include peer or utilization review components to identify and remedy deficiencies in quality. The program must have a mechanism for assessing its effectiveness and may measure care against preestablished standards.

Referral Form A form issued by the MCO that must be completed by the PCP to authorize a referral for a specialty service. The form may receive a number from the MCO, and requires the primary care physician to clearly delineate which services are authorized: the number of office visits, if lab tests or imaging can be ordered, and such.

Referral Fund A set amount of money set aside each month by the health plan. The monies in this fund are first used to pay for "referred" services such as specialty care or hospital services. Leftover funds may return to the health plan, or may be shared with the providers under a formula determined by the contract.

Risk The chance or possibility of loss. Risk is also defined in insurance terms as the possibility of loss associated with a given population.

Risk Pool A pool of money that is to be used for defined expenses. Commonly, if the money that is put at risk is not expended by the end of the year, some or all of it is returned to those managing the risk.

Staff Model HMO An HMO that delivers health services through a physician group that is controlled by the HMO unit; most physicians are salaried employees who deal exclusively with HMO members.

Self-Insurance The practice of an employer or organization assuming responsibility for healthcare losses of its employees. This usually includes setting up a fund against which claim payments are drawn and claims processing is often handled through an administrative services contract with an independent organization.

"Silent PPO" A PPO company that, rather than developing its own contracts with employers, the "silent PPO" simply utilizes the "assignment" clause of the provider contract and sells or leases the rights to the fee discounts to other health plans. This assignment occurs without the knowledge or consent of the provider, who had given up this right in the contract.

Stop Loss That point at which a third party has reinsurance to protect against the overly large single claim or the excessively high aggregate claim during a given period of time. Providers will buy stop loss insurance to protect themselves under capitated contracts.

Tertiary Care Subspecialty care usually requiring the facilities of a university affiliated or teaching hospital that has extensive diagnostic and treatment capabilities.

Third-Party Administrator (TPA) Company that contracts with employers who self-insure the healthcare benefits for their employees. The TPA develops and coordinates the self-insurance programs, processes and pays claims, and otherwise acts as an insurance carrier does. The TPA is paid an administrative fee by the employer.

Usual, Customary, and Reasonable (UCR) Health insurance plans that pay a physician's full charge if it is reasonable and does not exceed his or her usual charges and the amount customarily charged for the service by other physicians in the area.

Utilization Review (UR) Also known as utilization management or utilization control, utilization review is a systematic means for reviewing and controlling patients' use of medical care services as well as the appropriateness and quality of that care. Usually involves data collection, review and/or authorization, especially for services such as specialist referrals, emergency room use, and hospitalization.

Utilization The patterns of use of a service or type of service within a specified time. Utilization is usually expressed in rate per unit of population-at-risk for a given period (e.g., the number of hospital admissions per year per 1,000 persons enrolled in an HMO).

Withhold That portion of the fee, whether based upon fee for service or a capitation payment, that is withheld by an HMO to create an incentive for efficient care. The withheld funds are placed into a "risk pool." Based upon the performance of the members of the pool in terms of utilization of services as measured against a budget, some, all, or none of the funds are returned to the pool members after the end of the year.

APPENDIX F

Internet Web Sites for Medical Practice Management

AHCPR Agency for Healthcare Planning and Research (*www.ahcpr.gov*). Conquest 1.0 document in full can be downloaded.

AMA Online American Medical Association (*www.ama-assn.org*). Includes online text of JAMA and AMA News, publication catalogues, and Physician Insight searchable listing of 650,000 physicians.

CDC Online Centers for Disease Control (*www.cdc.gov*). Morbidity and Mortality Report Weekly Reports, data, hyperlinks.

Consumer Information Center (*www.pueblo.gsa.gov*). Download copy of many free and low cost Government Printing Office booklets at no charge. Many health education topics available.

Dilbert (*www.unitedmedia.com/comics/dilbert*). Fun.

HCFA Healthcare Financing Administration (*www.hcfa.gov*). Regulations, studies, data, access to Federal Register.

HCIA (*www.hcia.com*). Review summary descriptions of products. Extensive data sets.

Health Data National Health Information Resource Center (*www.nhirc.org*). Includes downloadable files of research and utilization data; other links.

HFMA Online Healthcare Financial Management Association (*www.hfma.org*). General information.

Journal of Nursing Jocularity (*www.jocularity.com*) Lots of fun. For people in the "business" only. The best since "House of God."

MEDACCESS (*www.medaccess.com*). Includes hospital locator search engine—by location, name, etc.

Medscape (*www.medscape.com*). Access to Medline; directed to clinicians.

MGMA Online Medical Group Management Association (*www.mgma.com*). Includes publications, several online discussion groups (must register—no fee).

Modern Healthcare Modern Healthcare magazine (*www.modernhealthcare.com*). Daily news summary Tuesday through Thursday.

NCQA National Committee for Quality Assurance (*www.ncqa.com*). Information, publications, full text of HEDIS 3.0.

PART - B News, Managed Care and Capitation Report (*www.ucg.com/health*). United Communications runs several excellent e-mail discussion groups that are actively used by participants.

SSA Online Social Security Administration (*www.ssa.gov*). Many online resources, including publications, copies of legislation, studies.

Your Health Daily (*www.nytsyn.com/med*). Daily news reports from Medical Tribune through the New York Times Syndication.

APPENDIX G

Information Resources

1. Healthcare Financial Management Association
   1-800-252-HFMA (4362)   www.hfma.org
   Books, self-study courses (including capitation)
   Managed Care Forum

2. Medical Group Management Association
   1-303-799-1111   www.mgma.com
   104 Inverness Terrace East
   Englewood, CO 80112-5306

Item 4893	Physician Incentive Plans (Search packet)
Item 4905	After the Contract: Operating the Practice Under Managed Care (search packet) Includes 80-page report: Living with Managed Care: A View From the Front
Item 4869	Cost Survey: 1996 Report Based on 1995 Data (book)
Item 4870	Physician Compensation and Production Survey: 1996 Report Based on 1995 Data (book)
Item 4951	Medical Group Practice Chart of Accounts (book)

3. American Medical Association
   1-800-621-8335   www.ama-assn.org
   American Medical News
   Books and publications, including CPT coding books

4. Irwin Professional Publishing
   1-800-634-3966   www.irwinpro.com
   Book publisher—co-publishes many titles with HFMA and MGMA
   Business Network Healthcare Seminars—one-day programs conducted all over the United States

Books:

Cherney, *The Capitation & Risk Sharing Guidebook*
Samuels, *Capitation: New Opportunities in Healthcare Delivery*
Todd, *The Managed Care Contracting Handbook: Planning and Negotiating the Managed Care Relationship*
Hekman, *Buying, Selling & Merging a Medical Practice: Proven Valuation and Negotiation Strategies*

ABOUT HFMA AND MGMA

HFMA is the nation's leading membership organization for more than 34,000 healthcare financial management professionals employed by hospitals, integrated delivery systems, managed care organizations, ambulatory and long-term care facilities, physician practices, accounting and consulting firms, and insurance agencies. Members' positions include chief financial officer, controller, patient accounts manager, accountant, and consultant. HFMA offers educational and professional development opportunities, information on key issues, technical data and networking opportunities, with the ultimate goal being to create a more supportive environment in which members do their business. For more information on HFMA call 1–800–252–HFMA (4362) extension 349.

MGMA is the leading professional membership association representing medical practice management. Today, MGMA's 6800 member organizations represent nearly two-thirds of all physicians involved in group practice in the United States. MGMA provides a variety of services to its organizational and individual members, including assistance in the areas of advocacy, communication, information, education, leadership and professional development, networking, and research. The services take a variety of forms, including publications, survey reports, an extensive library resource center, educational programs and conferences, representation in Washington, D.C., consulting services, comprehensive research, and professional certification.

For more information, write or call:

The Medical Group Management Association
104 Inverness Terrace East
Englewood, CO 80112–5306
(303) 799–1111

A Special Offer

The author publishes a newsletter, "Lucash Strategy Watch" commenting on business strategy in healthcare. Readers of this book can be placed on our mailing list and receive the next two issues with my compliments.

Please write:

Lucash Strategy Watch
Lucash & Company
1579-B Savannah Highway
Charleton, SC 29407

or email to: plucash@awod.com

For more information and discussion of the issues covered in this book, visit our web site: www.lucash.com

INDEX